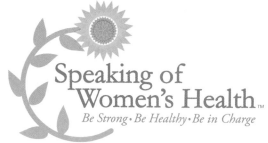

Speaking of
Women's Health™
Be Strong • Be Healthy • Be in Charge

IT'S THE
RIGHT
TIME

TO TAKE A PLEDGE
FOR BETTER HEALTH

THE BOOK
VOLUME IV

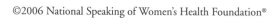

Table of Contents

The nutritional analysis provided is not intended for medical nutritional therapy. If you are following a strict diet for medical or dietary reasons, consult first with a physician or dietitian before planning your meals.

This book is designed to provide information about health, not medical advice. Please consult your physician if you have any questions or concerns.

Introduction

Every morning, upon waking, each of us is given a gift... a gift of 24 hours, 1,440 minutes and more than 86,000 seconds! Before jumping up to begin your rush to get out the door... take just one of those precious moments to think about how you will spend the rest of the day.

24 hours a day, 7 days a week, 52 weeks a year... today, tomorrow or next week... IT'S ALWAYS THE RIGHT TIME to make a change. That's what this book is all about... encouraging women to take time out for themselves and to focus on their own health... and, in the process, to help set an example for their loved ones. The key is to think in minutes, and not in hours or days or years. Small changes, done consistently, add up to improved *quality* of days, and increases the *quantity* of your weeks, months and years.

Here's something you can set your watch by... as you read through this book to educate yourself about your health, well-being and personal safety, you'll notice that every chapter is full of simple suggestions to help you achieve your best possible life! When you focus on eating a balanced, low-fat diet, rich in fruits and vegetables and strive for fun, physical activity on most days, you're off to a great start. Join your health care team, including your doctors, pharmacist and other trusted resources, so you can live the new **Speaking of Women's Health tagline: Be Strong • Be Healthy • Be In Charge.**

No matter what your age, health condition or level of fitness, it's never too late to make a fresh start. In fact, starting this very minute, **IT'S THE RIGHT TIME: To Take A Pledge For Better Health!**

The Staff at
Speaking of Women's Health

P.S. While you read this book, here's a fun challenge. Count the number of references to "time" in our chapters and recipes. E-mail us your guess for the total number of references to time by logging on to **www.speakingofwomenshealth.com.**

P.P.S. And, at Speaking of Women's Health, we knew it was THE RIGHT TIME to strengthen our logo! We think you'll agree... it's **Strong**, it's **Healthy**, it's **In Charge!**

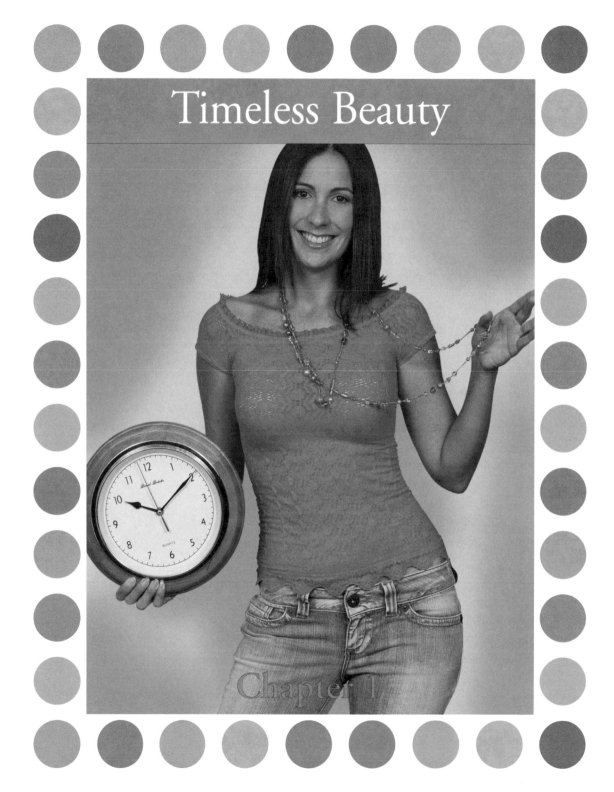

Timeless Beauty

Chapter 1

BEAUTY...

Pretty is what we can see on the surface...

Beauty is what lies within all of us

There is the obvious beauty – what is visible on the surface... your appearance. There is the beauty that is unseen, which comes from within and radiates outward.

Have you ever looked at someone and noticed that they have that special glow about them? You couldn't pinpoint whether it was their hair, skin, outfit or, personality, but they had that special something. What is it that makes them so alluring?

Beauty is more than what we look like. Some people may define beauty as an actress at the Oscars in her stunning gown, or it could be that action hero on the big screen that takes another person's breath away. In reality, beauty is what appeals to our hearts. Beauty begins from within. As we often say, beauty is the reflection of one's inner spirit. In a recent study, a spirit full of zest, a passion for life and a healthy dose of self-confidence were ranked as 3 of the highest qualities that men found "sexy" in a woman. In addition to a woman's physique, half of those surveyed said that a woman's smile was the first thing they noticed. And... we'd like to add that a smile is contagious. When you smile at someone, they can't help but smile back at you.

Now, the $64,000 question is... how do you achieve that level of confidence and self-esteem? Part of it certainly comes from what we see when we look in the mirror.

And, if we look good, we feel good. When we feel good, we take better care of ourselves. Looking good is one thing; feeling good is everything! That is healthy living. Beauty is a combination of inner feelings and an outward glow. Every woman can shine, but sometimes she needs a little help!

*In the mornin',
in the evenin'...
you've got the time.*

*It's essential
to develop a skincare
routine that is
simple and do-able.
Beautiful skin is
healthy skin.*

*Here's a routine you
can set your clock by:*

✔ *Cleanse*
✔ *Tone*
✔ *Moisturize*
✔ *Protect*

Beauty is More Than Skin Deep

This is a phrase that everyone has heard and it's true. But, did you know that your skin is the body's largest organ? It comprises 15–20% of your total weight. As the largest organ that everyone can see, it's important that it is taken care of properly.

Your skin is more than an outer shell; it's an indicator of the state of your health and reveals the story of your life. Your skin speaks volumes.

The skin provides the following:

Protection – The skin serves as a barrier from infection, pollution, trauma and the elements.

Hydration – Skin locks in the body's moisture. This is why you are advised to apply moisturizer after you bathe or wash your face, while your skin is still damp.

Regulation of Body Temperature – A considerable amount of heat is lost through the skin. Even under conditions of heat or exercise, the body temperature usually remains almost normal.

Excretion – The skin sweats to cool the body when it is hot and conserves heat when it is cold. In addition, small amounts of waste are excreted through perspiration.

Sense of Touch – There are many nerve endings in the skin that allow us to feel pleasure and pain, pressure and temperature.

Production of Vitamin D – Our skin's exposure to sunlight alters a substance in the skin, allowing Vitamin D to be produced. Vitamin D is necessary for the body's proper absorption of calcium and phosphates from food.

A Wrinkle in Time

As we age, our skin's cells do not have as rapid a turnover as they did when we were younger. With this slower cell replacement, our skin may start to have dullness to it and the texture may appear different. The collagen and elastin fibers that provide the supporting structure for the skin start to weaken and unravel so that the skin's elasticity diminishes. All of these changes are compounded by gravity, which may result in fine lines, wrinkles, droopy eyelids and jowls.

Although the sun causes most skin damage attributed to premature aging, even people who avoid the sun will notice changes occurring. **The good news is...** with good skincare and the availability of high quality skincare products, you can keep your skin vitalized.

Here are some important tips to remember. To look good on the outside, you have to take care of yourself on the inside. Remember the following:

✔ Drink plenty of water.

✔ Take care of your face and neck...but, don't forget the rest of your body! Use moisturizing body wash and lotions to help keep your skin glowing.

✔ Get plenty of rest.

✔ Protect with sunscreen before going out in the sun to help protect your skin from the sun's harmful rays – the number one cause of premature aging. Use products that have a Sun Protection Factor (SPF) of 15 or higher.

✔ Avoid mid-day sun between 10 a.m. – 3 p.m.

✔ Avoid tanning beds. Get with the times... If you can't resist that "just off the beach" glow, try a sunless tanning product. Today, you have many options, whether you're looking for just a blush of color or a bronzed look overall.

✔ Check your skin often for signs of skin cancer. If you see changes, call your doctor right away. (For danger signs, see www.speakingofwomenshealth.com)

✔ Eat a balanced diet and exercise regularly.

✔ Stop smoking. It is known that smoking is damaging to delicate skin, especially around the mouth and eyes.

✔ Choose products that are specially-formulated to work best for your skin type. Today's skincare products and cosmetics can be found for normal, dry, oily or sensitive skin; but, that's not all! Choose from anti-aging products that minimize fine lines and wrinkles, anti-acne to help minimize pores and hypoallergenic for sensitive skin.

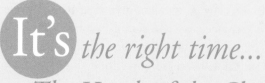

It's *the right time...*
The Hands of the Clock Go 'Round

Take a Minute... Test Your Beauty IQ

Question: Will a toner dry out my skin?

Answer: No. Alcohol-free toners are very gentle and are an important part of your daily skincare routine. They will minimize the appearance of pores, restore the natural pH balance of your skin and remove any traces of makeup and dirt. Do not confuse toners with astringents, which contain alcohol and are meant to be drying for very oily skin.

Question: Is there a difference between eye creams and other moisturizers?

Answer: Yes. Eye creams are formulated specifically for your eye's delicate skin area, which has no oil beds and requires special care.

Question: Does the sun play a big role in the health of my skin?

Answer: You bet it does! Approximately 90% of your skin's aging is due to sun exposure. Always remember to wear a sunscreen under your makeup. Some moisturizers even contain a Sun Protection Factor (SPF). If you want that "golden look," try sunless tanners or bronzers.

Question: Do I really need to use an eye makeup remover to remove my shadow, liner and mascara?

Answer: Yes. The skin around your eye is very delicate. You do not want to use anything oily or harsh. Apply your remover to a cotton round/pad and hold on your eyelid for several seconds. Then wipe gently downward. Now you are ready to cleanse your face.

Question: When coloring my hair at home, what can I do to touchup the roots?

Answer: First, always follow the instructions on the hair color box! Then, begin by applying some of the product to the roots only. Leave this on for the amount of time recommended in the directions. Apply the remaining hair color to the previously colored part of your hair for the last 5 minutes of processing only. This will refresh your color and make it as vibrant as the newly-colored growth.

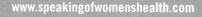

Question: What are the advantages of a lip liner?

Answer: A lip liner will provide definition to your lip shape. It also prevents feathering and bleeding of your lipstick, by acting as a "fence" to keep the lipstick in place.

Question: How should I choose a blush?

Answer: There are 2 main criteria when selecting blush – type and color. If you apply blush over a powdered face, then you should select a powder blush. If you apply blush over your liquid makeup or on freshly-moisturized skin, then select a creamy blush. Because common forms bond best, the application will be easier and the product will last longer. For a professional look, it's best to match the color of your blush to the color of your lipstick. Now's a great time to have some fun with shimmering shades and bronzers.

Question: Does eyeliner look better when applied to the top lid, the bottom lid or both?

Answer: There is no right or wrong answer. Cosmetics are meant to enhance your natural beauty. So, try a few "looks" and select the one that suits you best. If your intent is to make your eyes look bigger, do not line both the top and bottom – that will make your eyes look smaller.

Question: Any secrets to good mascara application?

Answer: Of course! Always position the brush/comb as close to the base of the eyelash as possible and then sweep outward. Start by coating the top of the lashes on your upper eyelid. Then coat the bottom of those top lashes. Apply a few extra coats to the lashes on the outer end of the eye to really extend the lash line. Then apply several coats to the lashes on your lower lid to really make them noticeable. Do not allow the mascara to dry in between coats.

Question: I'm too busy to apply lots of makeup. What can I do to look beautiful?

Answer: The "beauty basics" are things that we all can do. Eat healthy. Drink lots of water. Get 8 hours of sleep a night. Try to minimize stress. If you add a few simple practices, such as daily cleansing, toning and moisturizing... and protection of your skin... you will look truly beautiful!

Just as dry winter air can wreak havoc on your hair, so does your summer air conditioner. Counteract the drying effects with a humidifier, which puts water back into the air and helps your hair (and skin) stay moisturized, and look more youthful.

Time… "Hair's" the Long and Short of It!

Shopping for (and trying out) the right shampoo, conditioner and styling products can be a day of fun. Shiny, healthy and well-groomed hair will ensure your sense of vitality. Also, consider using a good hair stylist. There is nothing like a new haircut to make a difference. A cut with diagonal lines that "lift" and draw attention away from the jaw line can do wonders for your new look. Whatever style you choose, get it trimmed regularly to maintain its health. And, just as your skin needs proper care – so does your hair. Choose a shampoo that meets your needs, your lifestyle and is formulated for your hair type.

In this day and age of soft hair color choices and highlights or lowlights, a woman does not have to live with gray hair unless it is flattering. **The good news is…** there are many choices you can try at home to update your look. Try highlights to your existing color to lift and focus attention above the brow line. Use lowlights to tone down your existing color, which makes for a natural look. Many of today's products for home are enriched with natural ingredients to protect and nurture your hair while you color.

Pay close attention to your hair and listen to its needs. If you notice a change in texture or condition, take time to evaluate what may be happening and make adjustments. Your hair, like your body, sends you signals about what it needs. Is it drier, oilier or frizzier? Get to know your hair and look for products that meet its needs.

Pamper your hair at least once a week. This can be as simple as giving yourself a hot oil treatment, a relaxing scalp massage or applying a special deep conditioning pack. Do something for your hair that makes it feel special. Your hair will respond in kind.

Time to Restart the Clock With a Mini-Makeover?

Some of us have had the same hairstyle and worn the same makeup for years because we're afraid to try something new. We can't part with our long hair or we're intimidated by a change in color. Give yourself a makeover this weekend! Here's how...

✔ Find out what haircut best suits your face shape.

✔ Look in magazines for styles you like.

✔ Always take pictures with you to the salon.

✔ Show and tell. Sit down with the stylist before you get your hair wet, and show him or her exactly how short you're comfortable going. Pointing out with your hands says much more than stating, "a couple inches." If you are feeling brave, than tell your stylist you're comfortable with change and willing to let her work her magic. Be sure to discuss your lifestyle with your stylist. If you're not willing to spend more than 15 minutes per day styling your hair, be sure to point this out before you get a cut that may require more.

✔ Consider color. If you have dark hair, try going a shade lighter or try out a deep auburn. If you have lighter hair, go for highlights.

✔ Stop by your local store and get new makeup. Treat yourself to a new blush, a new eye shadow shade or a new lipstick to make your cheeks, eyes or lips fabulous! As the seasons change, experiment with new shades or colors. Spend a little time on yourself... you're worth it!

✔ Don't forget your nails... an at-home manicure and/or pedicure can really make you feel special. Soak your feet while you work on your nails, or read a good book! Relax, enjoy... PAMPER!!!

✔ Go out for dinner with friends or your family and celebrate your new look!

Take a Break!

You know that a high stress level is bad for your mood... did you know it also affects your skin? Treat yourself to at least one relaxing, pampering activity per week, be it a bubble bath surrounded by glowing candles, a facial or a movie rental marathon at home.

Pretty is as pretty does…and it comes from the inside. We just spent a few minutes talking about your outer appearance, now, let's focus on your inner sense of beauty. Your self-esteem can be made up of how you see life, as well as how you see yourself. According to Nancy Coey, Speaking of Women's Health presenter, a good start is "Finding Gifts in Everyday Life."

✔ Know that gifts always surround you. From the joy of waking up every morning, to the small ways your loved ones show they care.

✔ "You have to be present to win" is true for door prizes… and for life. Being an active participant in your life is the only way to live it fully and most enjoyably.

✔ The vast majority of what we worry about never happens. Concentrate on the parts of your life that you can change, in a positive way… and make that change stick!

✔ Look for the good, and train your eyes, by keeping a "Best Thing of the Day" journal. This will help you see the positive… and the gifts that life brings… in any situation!

✔ If you train your eyes, you can change your life. When you teach your eyes to look for good, they inevitably find it!

✔ Let go of what doesn't matter. Dwelling on the past is ineffective… so start thinking about the positive things in your future!

✔ It truly is better to give… try and experience its power!

✔ Open yourself to lessons from unlikely teachers.

✔ Find teachers… even in unlikely places.

✔ Harness the power inherent in small things.

Your Time to Shine!

Nothing celebrates your inner beauty more than a beautiful smile. As we've said, the first thing that most of us notice, when having a conversation with someone, is their smile. Healthy, bright white teeth and a nice smile always catch the attention of onlookers.

To make your teeth white and healthy, eat a healthy diet. Brushing your teeth after every meal is also a good idea. There are whitening toothpastes, mouthwashes and strips available at your local store that you can try as well. If you are facing any problems or difficulties with your teeth, don't wait too long to see your dentist. And, be sure to visit your dentist twice a year for healthy teeth and gums.

Your smile is your gift to the world... share it often! It's something you can give away as often as you like and you'll never run out.

Speaking of Women's Health dental expert, Jordan Pelchovitz, DDS, suggests the following tips:

✔ Switch to an electric toothbrush. These newer brushes do a great job of cleaning your teeth, gums and tongue, and some have a timer to allow for adequate cleaning time.

✔ Floss at least once daily. Ask your dentist or hygienist to show you the proper way to make sure you are getting your gums and teeth as clean as possible.

✔ If you can't brush after a meal or snack, chew gum that contains the sugar-substitute xylitol. It helps fight decay by producing saliva, your body's natural tooth cleanser.

✔ Avoid tobacco products in any form. They can cause staining of the teeth, gum disease and cancer of the mouth and throat.

✔ Eat a balanced diet. The Vitamin C in fruits and vegetables help promote healthy gums by maintaining collagen levels. Foods like milk, yogurt and cottage cheese bathe the teeth in calcium, which helps fight tooth decay.

✔ Consider protecting against bone loss with dental implants when you lose a tooth. An implant maintains the bones that support your other teeth, lips and cheeks.

✔ Straight teeth are the easiest to keep clean and free of decay and gum disease. Ask your dentist if you are a candidate for invisible braces, so you will not have traditional metal braces.

✔ Do not ignore gums that bleed during brushing and flossing. Bleeding may be a sign of gum disease, which has been linked to heart disease, osteoporosis and diabetes.

✔ Hormones affect your mouth just as they do the rest of your body. Estrogen levels during puberty, menstruation, pregnancy and menopause fluctuate, which can cause gum disease.

✔ Preventive care is the best care. See your dentist every 6 months for a thorough cleaning, oral cancer screening and x-rays to detect problems early, when they are the easiest (and least costly) to fix.

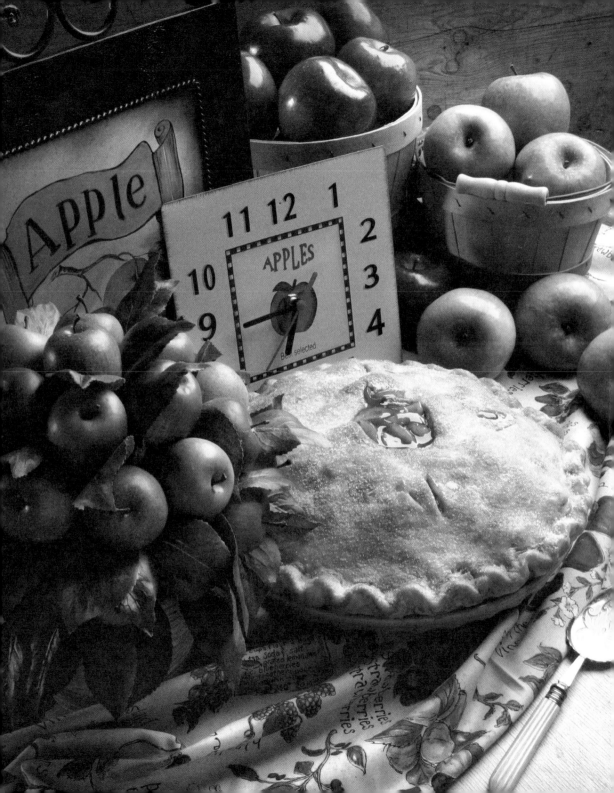

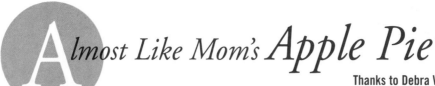

Almost Like Mom's *Apple Pie*

Thanks to Debra Warner
Buyer, Wal-Mart

Take a little time to make this, and you'll be the apple of someone's eye.
It's a reduced-calorie, "sweetie pie" of a recipe.

INGREDIENTS

Filling

6 oz.	frozen unsweetened apple juice concentrate
2½ Tbsp.	all-purpose flour
1 tsp.	cinnamon
¼ tsp.	salt
6	medium apples, sliced. Try different varieties for different flavor (leave peel on for added nutritional value).
1 Tbsp.	heart-healthy buttery spread
½ tsp.	nutmeg

Crust

2 cups	all-purpose flour
¼ tsp.	salt
½ cup	canola oil
⅓ cup	plus a few tablespoons well-chilled non-fat milk

NUTRITIONAL ANALYSIS
Servings per recipe: 8
Each serving contains approximately:

368	calories
4 g.	protein
51 g.	carbohydrates
6 g.	fat (1 g. saturated fat)

PREPARATION

Filling

- Preheat oven to 450 degrees. In a small saucepan, combine the frozen apple juice, flour, cinnamon and salt. Stir constantly over medium heat until the mixture is thick and bubbly, 3–5 minutes. Peel and slice the apples and stir them into the apple juice mixture. Pour the mixture into the unbaked pie shell and dot with buttery spread. Position the top crust over the filling, cutting slits for the steam to escape. Trim and seal the edges. Brush the top very lightly with water and sprinkle with nutmeg if desired. Bake at 450 degrees for 15 minutes. Reduce heat to 350 degrees and bake for 30 minutes more.

Crust

- For crust, combine flour and salt in bowl. Combine oil and milk in a covered jar and shake vigorously to mix. Make a well in the center of flour mixture and pour in the oil and milk mixture. Using a pastry blender or working with your fingertips, form a ball. Don't over-work. Divide into 2 balls, one slightly larger than the other. Roll out the larger one between 2 sheets of plastic wrap so it is just large enough to cover the bottom and sides of a 9-inch pie pan. Roll out the smaller ball for the top.

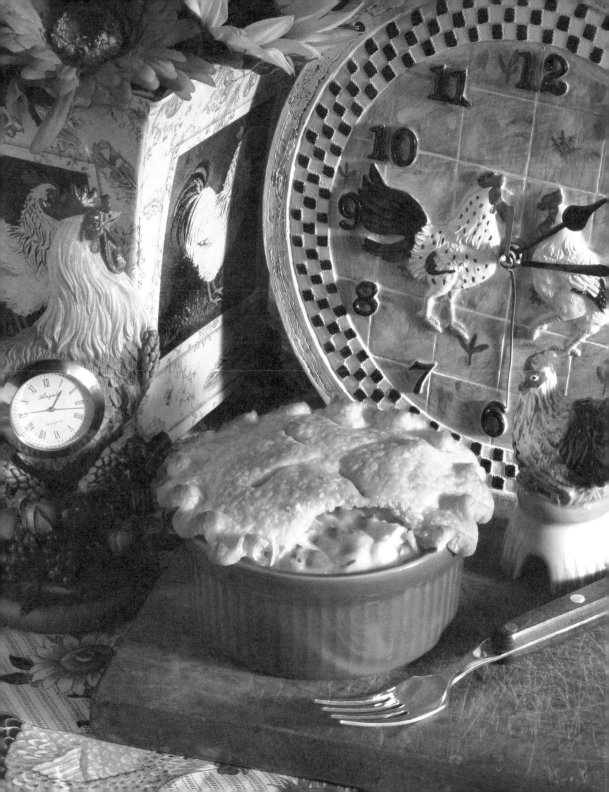

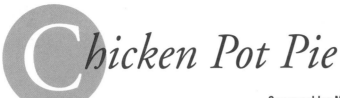

Chicken Pot Pie

**Thanks to Jennifer Williams
Consumables Marketing Manager, Wal-Mart**

No need for the dinner bell... your chicks, and even your rooster, will scurry to the kitchen when the aroma of this chicken pot pie fills the room at dinner time.

INGREDIENTS

Filling

2 cups	low-sodium, non-fat chicken broth
1 cup	chopped onion
½ lb.	new potatoes, unpeeled and diced
½ tsp.	dried thyme
¼ cup	cornstarch
1 cup	non-fat milk
2 cups	diced assorted vegetables – choose from zucchini, yellow squash, green bell pepper, red bell pepper, carrots, celery, peas... any of your favorites!
1 cup	sliced mushrooms
1 tsp.	Dijon mustard
2 cups	diced, cooked chicken breast
	salt & pepper to taste

Topping

Use recipe for crust on page 15, cut in half.

NUTRITIONAL ANALYSIS
Servings per recipe: 6
Each serving contains approximately:
- 314 calories
- 22 g. protein
- 36 g. carbohydrates
- 10 g. fat (3 g. saturated fat)

PREPARATION

Filling

- Preheat oven to 400 degrees. Bring 1 cup broth to a boil in a large pot. Add onion and cook 3 minutes, until soft, then add remaining 1 cup broth, potatoes and thyme. Bring to a boil and cook until potatoes are tender. Add zucchini, yellow squash, red and green peppers, mushrooms, salt and pepper for the last minute. Meanwhile, combine cornstarch and milk and stir until smooth, add mustard. Bring to a boil and cook 5 minutes. Stir in chicken and remove from heat. Pour into one 9-inch deep-dish pie plate, or divide into 6 individual smaller dishes.

Topping

- Roll crust into circle large enough to cover 9-inch pie plate or individual ramekins. Cover filling and pinch edges to side of pan. Cut vents into top and bake 20 minutes, or until top is golden.

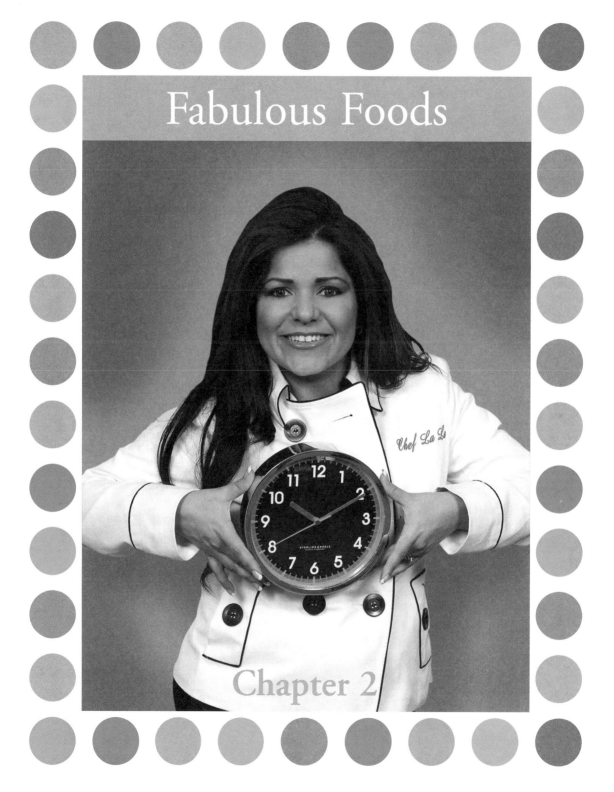

Fabulous Foods

Chapter 2

IT'S TIME TO EAT RIGHT...

Nutrition for a healthy lifestyle!

It may seem obvious, but eating right is one of the first steps in living a healthy life. Our diet provides the nutrients and energy we need to survive, so choosing the right foods is essential. Proper nutrition includes a balance between what is "good for you" and what "tastes good." **The good news is...** the two can easily go hand-in-hand. Nature has graciously supplied us with plentiful options for optimal nutrition.

In nearly every chapter of this book, we highlight recommendations for improving your health by improving your diet and combining that with daily physical activity. Believe it or not, the types of food you eat actually DO help control your health and how you look. Staying healthy means eating nutritiously. It's important to choose foods that are full of nutrients, and rich in vitamins and minerals. We all want to live longer, feel better and look good. And, to improve our longevity, we need to watch what and how much we eat every day.

In addition to choosing healthy foods, balance and moderation are the keys to successful eating. The "key 3" for a healthy diet include: controlling portions, limiting fats and sugars and choosing a variety of foods, including fruits, vegetables, whole grains and lean protein, in your meals (see Food Pyramid on page 20). You may find it helpful to eat a combination of 5 or 6 smaller meals or healthy snacks, as opposed to 3 large meals. Many nutritionists are now recommending this.

So, for a healthy diet you can set your watch by... read on! And, don't be alarmed... it can be simple to fill your hours with nutritious, great-tasting foods!

The Food Guide Pyramid

Most experts agree that the average woman requires about 2,000 calories each day. Your diet should be balanced and contain the appropriate amount of calories and nutrients. The National Food Guide Pyramid states that, as a general rule of thumb, most people need the amounts from each food group below.

GRAINS – Make half your grains whole: Eat at least 3 oz. of whole-grain cereals, breads, crackers, rice or pasta every day. 1 oz. is about 1 slice of whole-grain bread, about 1 cup of breakfast cereal, or ½ cup of cooked brown rice, cereal or pasta. Of your total of 6 oz. every day, make 3 oz. whole-grains.

VEGETABLES – Vary your veggies: Eat dark-green veggies like broccoli, spinach and other dark leafy greens. Include orange vegetables like carrots and sweet potatoes. Choose dry beans and peas including pinto beans, garbanzo beans, kidney beans and lentils. Eat 2½ cups of vegetables every day.

FRUITS – Focus on fruits: Eat a variety of fruit. Choose fresh, frozen, canned or dried fruit. Eat 2 cups of fruit every day. ***Nutritionists now suggest eating 7–9 servings of fruits and vegetables every day.***

MILK – Get your calcium-rich foods: Go low-fat or fat-free when you choose milk, yogurt and other dairy products. If you don't or can't consume milk, choose lactose-free products or other calcium sources such as fortified foods and beverages. Get 3 cups every day; for kids aged 2–8, it's 2 cups a day.

MEATS & BEANS – Go lean with protein: Choose low-fat or lean meats and poultry. Bake it, broil it or grill it. Vary your protein routine – choose more fish, beans, peas, nuts and seeds. Eat 5½ oz. every day. (NOTE: Speaking of Women's Health keynote speaker, Zonya Foco, RD, LD, recommends choosing meats that say "loin," as in tenderloin, sirloin, ground loin and pork loin.)

Food for Thought

Did you know that there are foods you eat daily that are beneficial for improving digestion, preventing cardiovascular disease, enhancing weight loss and supporting urinary function? Our expert, Rita Heikenfeld, RD, suggests the following "Super Foods for Women."

- ✔ **"C" yourself healthy.** Water is the best health drink and a splash of lemon juice in it provides Vitamin C, which helps your body absorb iron and calcium and is a gentle liver cleanser.

- ✔ **"Flax your muscles!"** A great source of Omega-3s, protein and fiber, flax is great for your hair, skin, nails, eyes and brain.

- ✔ **Shake, shake, shake... your cinnamon!** Yes, on almost everything. This helps lower cholesterol and improves glucose levels.

- ✔ **Bone-building calcium** in yogurt also helps keep your intestinal tract healthy.

- ✔ **Health from the deep... seafood!** Coral-colored salmon and other coldwater fish may help reduce the risk of heart disease, breast and colon cancers.

- ✔ **Go for the grains!** Whole wheat, brown rice, barley and oats are powerhouse sources of complex carbs for long-lasting energy.

- ✔ **Lean on legumes.** Lentils, beans and other legumes are low in fat and high in protein, fiber and vitamins and minerals. These good carbs can send cholesterol south and help keep blood sugar steady.

- ✔ **Nuts about nuts!** Full of fiber, protein and mainly good fats, nuts contain Vitamin E, heart-healthy copper and magnesium. Almonds contain calcium, and walnuts have Omega-3s.

Don't Snooze Through Breakfast...

Jump start your mornings. Breakfast is considered the most important meal of the day. Each morning, we need to fuel our bodies so they work properly. Yet, many of us don't allot enough time in the morning to enjoy a proper breakfast.

It's *the right time...*

"Hour" Recipe for a Healthy Diet...
Balance Your Plate With Variety

It is important to know and understand how foods are broken down. Make sure you eat a variety of food for a healthy diet.

CARBOHYDRATES are your body's main energy source. Complex carbs include legumes, grains and starchy vegetables such as potatoes, peas and corn. Simple carbs, also called sugars, are found mainly in fruits and milk, as well as in foods made with sugar, such as candy and other sweets.

Recommendation: Get 45–65% of your daily calories, at least 130 grams a day, from carbohydrates. Emphasize complex carbs, especially from whole grains and beans, and nutrient-rich fruits and milk. Limit sugars from candy and other sweets.

PROTEIN is essential to human life. Your skin, bones, muscles and organ tissue all contain protein. It's found in your blood, hormones and enzymes, too. Protein is found in many plant foods, as well as from animal sources. Legumes, nuts, seeds, poultry, seafood, meat and dairy products are your richest sources of protein.

Recommendation: Between 10–35% of your total daily calories, at least 46 grams a day for women, can come from protein.

FIBER is the part of plant foods that your body doesn't digest and absorb. There are 2 basic types: soluble and insoluble. Insoluble fiber adds bulk to your stool and can help prevent constipation. Vegetables, wheat bran and other whole grains are good sources of insoluble fiber. Soluble fiber may help improve your cholesterol and blood sugar levels. Oats, dried beans and some fruits, such as apples and oranges, are good sources of soluble fiber.

Recommendation: Get 25–35 grams of fiber in your diet every day. Fiber is an essential part of a healthy diet and is key to digestive tract health.

CHOLESTEROL can be confusing. It is vital to the structure and function of all your cells, but it's also the main substance in fatty deposits (plaques) that can develop in your arteries. *Healthy bodies make all of the cholesterol they need for cell function.* That is why monitoring your diet is essential. Animal foods, such as meat, poultry, seafood, eggs, dairy products and butter all contain amounts of cholesterol. See Chapter 4 for more information on good and bad cholesterol.

Recommendation: Limit your intake of cholesterol to no more than 200 milligrams a day.

FATS help your body absorb many essential vitamins, maintain the structure and function of cell membranes, and boost your immune system. But fat is a very concentrated energy source, providing twice as many calories per gram as carbohydrates and protein. And too much of certain types of fat, such as saturated fat and trans fat, can increase your blood cholesterol levels and your risk of coronary artery disease.

Recommendation: Limit total fat (saturated and unsaturated) to no more than 30% of your daily calories. Emphasize fats from healthier sources, such as nuts and olive, canola and peanut oils.

SATURATED FAT is most often found in animal products, such as red meat, poultry, butter and whole milk. Other foods high in saturated fat include coconut, palm and other tropical oils. Saturated fat is the main dietary culprit in raising your blood cholesterol and increasing your risk of coronary artery disease.

Recommendation: Limit your daily intake of saturated fat to no more than 7–10% of your total calories. For most women, this means no more than 20 grams a day.

The REALLY GOOD NEWS IS...

An increasing body of scientific research suggests that specific compounds found in cocoa may have health benefits.

Research has shown that certain types of specially-processed dark chocolate can retain cocoa flavanols. These compounds are similar to those found in red wines and green tea. Research on these naturally occurring flavanols is showing great promise in maintaining heart health by helping to promote healthy circulation.

So... when you're craving chocolate, choose dark chocolate and enjoy in moderation.

"Weight" a Minute

If you are like many women, you may find yourself consumed by the numbers on the scale. The truth is that we need to focus more on a healthy weight than on a particular number. So many women are busy with day-to-day activities, that it is tempting to grab something unhealthy to eat on-the-go. But remember, what you feed your body does help determine how you look.

Fortunately, today you have options. These include liquid meal replacements that may help manage your weight. Other options include healthy cereal and snack bars. With just a bit of planning, you can grab these healthy alternatives from your desk, car, purse or backpack. When you choose to eat healthy, incorporating balanced meals and healthy snacking, you will be more successful in maintaining a healthy weight for your body.

Good Tips for Controlling Calories:

✔ Keep a food diary for a week, writing down everything that you eat and drink. People who are overweight often don't realize how much they are eating.

✔ Use your food diary to find ways of cutting down calories. For instance, you could cut 500 calories per day by changing the balance of foods on your plate; less cheese and more salad with your dinner. Or, you could cut out a regular snack food and replace it with a piece of fruit.

✔ Don't forget that drinks count toward your daily calorie intake. Alcohol is high in calories – 3 beers could add up to 600 calories. Some juices, regular sodas and coffee drinks have lots of sugar. If you need to limit your sugar intake, consider treating yourself to zero-calorie, zero-sodium, zero-caffeine options.

Nutrition and Diabetes

The Not-So-Sweet Truth about Blood Sugar

Because diabetes is such a national epidemic and because it causes such serious health issues, we want to talk about prevention, detection and treatment. Diabetes is a disease of the pancreas, an organ behind your stomach that produces the hormone insulin. Insulin helps the body use food for energy. When a person has diabetes, the pancreas either cannot produce enough insulin, uses the insulin incorrectly, or both. Insulin works together with glucose in the bloodstream to help it enter the body's cells to be burned for energy. If the insulin isn't functioning properly, glucose cannot enter the cells. This causes glucose levels in the blood to rise, creating a condition of high blood sugar or diabetes, and leaving the cells without fuel.

What Causes Diabetes?

Health care providers do not yet know what causes diabetes. The following factors may increase your chance of getting diabetes:

✔ Family history of diabetes or inherited tendency

✔ African-American, Hispanic or Native-American race or ethnic descent

✔ Obesity (being 20% or more above your appropriate body weight)

✔ Physical stress (such as surgery or illness)

✔ Use of certain medications

✔ Injury to pancreas (such as infection, tumor, surgery or accident)

✔ Auto-immune disease

✔ Hypertension

✔ Abnormal blood cholesterol or triglyceride levels

✔ Age (risk increases with age)

✔ Alcohol use (risk increases with years of heavy alcohol use)

✔ Smoking

✔ Pregnancy (Pregnancy puts extra stress on a woman's body, which causes some women to develop gestational diabetes. Blood sugar levels often return to normal after childbirth. Yet, women who develop diabetes during pregnancy have an increased chance of developing diabetes later in life.)

What are the Symptoms of Diabetes?

These symptoms may include:

- ✔ Increased thirst
- ✔ Frequent urination
- ✔ Fatigue (weak, tired feeling)
- ✔ Increased hunger (especially after eating)
- ✔ Unexplained weight loss or gain
- ✔ Numbness or tingling of the hands or feet

- ✔ Dry mouth
- ✔ Blurred vision
- ✔ Loss of consciousness (rare)
- ✔ Sores that heal slowly
- ✔ Dry, itchy skin

You hold the key to managing your diabetes by doing the following, according to Janet Bohne, RD, LD; Lea Ann Dick, RD, LD, CDE and Rita Gattermeyer, RN:

- ✔ **Find Out.** Know your blood glucose results. A simple screening test can determine if you already have diabetes or symptoms of pre-diabetes. (See Chapter 4)
- ✔ **Take Charge.** Keep track of blood pressure readings and cholesterol levels.
- ✔ **Take Care.** Spend time on your own health. It will allow you to be able to take better care of others in your life.
- ✔ **Get Moving!** Reduce your risk for developing diabetes by increasing your physical activity. Find something you enjoy doing and move your body every day.
- ✔ **Say "Yes" to Healthy Eating!** Diets come and go, but the weight often stays. Healthy eating is about daily balance and moderation, not about restriction.
- ✔ **Listen Up!** Listen to your body. Learn to eat when you're hungry, and stop when you're satisfied. No need to always "clean your plate."
- ✔ **Relax.** Find ways to cope with stress besides eating.
- ✔ **Eat Your Veggies!** Nature's bounty provides important nutrients with very few calories.
- ✔ **Go Nuts!** Try a handful of walnuts or almonds each day to get some healthy fats in your diet.
- ✔ **Spice Up Your Life!** Add a sprinkling of cinnamon to your hot tea, coffee or toast each day to improve your body's ability to use insulin.

TIMELY TIPS
for Healthy Eating

✔ **Eat a rainbow of colors.** The more intense the colors of your fruits and vegetables, the more vitamins, minerals and antioxidants they provide. To name a few, think of tomatoes, dark leafy greens, carrots and berries.

✔ **Watch serving sizes.** "Super sizing" does not mean "super nutrition." For example, the typical bagel today is actually equivalent to 4 slices of bread. An appropriate serving of meat (3 oz.) is the size of a deck of cards.

✔ **Avoid skipping meals.** Skipping meals may lower your metabolism and cause you to over-eat at other times. It's not "no" snacks, it's "know" snacks.

✔ **When dining out, leave your "party hat" mentality at home.** Every time you eat out does not have to be a party!

✔ **Think about your food choices over the day... make trade-offs.** For example, if your restaurant meal will be high in calories or fat, eat foods with less calories or fat at the other meals.

✔ **Become a savvy restaurant consumer.** Be assertive but not aggressive. Pretend the restaurant is providing you with your own personal chef. Most restaurants are more than willing to work with you to keep you happy (and healthy)!

✔ **Remember, a variety of food and fitness is the Spice of Life.** Look to the Food Pyramid on page 20 for guidance. All food groups are essential for good health.

Facts about Colon Cancer

All adults are at risk for GI problems, and the risk increases as we get older. It is estimated that colon cancer will strike 1 in 20 people during their lifetime.

Fiber is important to digestive tract health.

✔ *Get a colonoscopy if you are over age 50! Colon cancer is treatable if detected early.*

✔ *Seeing red is not good! Rectal bleeding is NEVER normal and should always be evaluated.*

✔ *Know your family history. Talk to your health care provider for earlier screenings if you are at risk.*

✔ *Colon cancer screenings save lives! Do not be embarrassed to get screened.*

✔ *Do not be afraid to ask your doctor hard questions! You are placing your life in their hands.*

"Procrastination is the thief of time."

—Edward Young

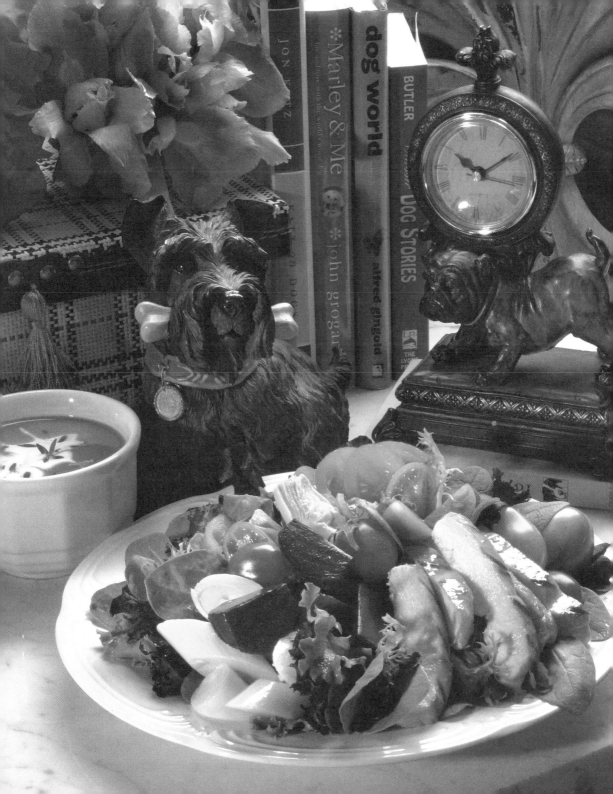

California Salad

Thanks to Clara Aquilar
Spanish Card Marketing, American Greetings

Cool off during the dog days of summer with this refreshing California Salad. Add our super soup, made with red peppers and tomatoes, as another tasty treat. This recipe will make you sit up and beg for more!

INGREDIENTS

2	boneless, skinless chicken breast halves
½ cup	olive oil
¼ cup	lemon juice
1	garlic clove, minced
	Kosher salt and freshly ground black pepper, to taste
4 cups	mixed salad greens (choose arugula, radicchio, spinach, romaine)
1 can	artichoke hearts
1 can	hearts of palm
½ cup each	red and yellow grape tomatoes
1 can	whole baby beets
¼ cup	fat-free feta cheese

Dressing

½ cup	olive oil
¼ cup	lemon juice
2 tsp.	Dijon mustard
2 Tbsp.	balsamic vinegar

PREPARATION

- Marinate chicken breast in olive oil, lemon juice, garlic clove, salt & pepper. Marinate 2–4 hours.
- Grill chicken until the juices run clear.
- Arrange greens into individual dishes, divided into 1 cup greens per person. Arrange artichoke hearts, hearts of palm, tomatoes and beets. Sprinkle with feta cheese.

Dressing

- Mix all ingredients together and shake well before serving.

Log on to *www.speakingofwomenshealth.com* for a zesty Roasted Red Pepper soup recipe to accompany the California Salad.

NUTRITIONAL ANALYSIS
Servings per recipe: 4
Each serving contains approximately:

277	calories
42 g.	protein
15 g.	carbohydrates
6 g.	fat

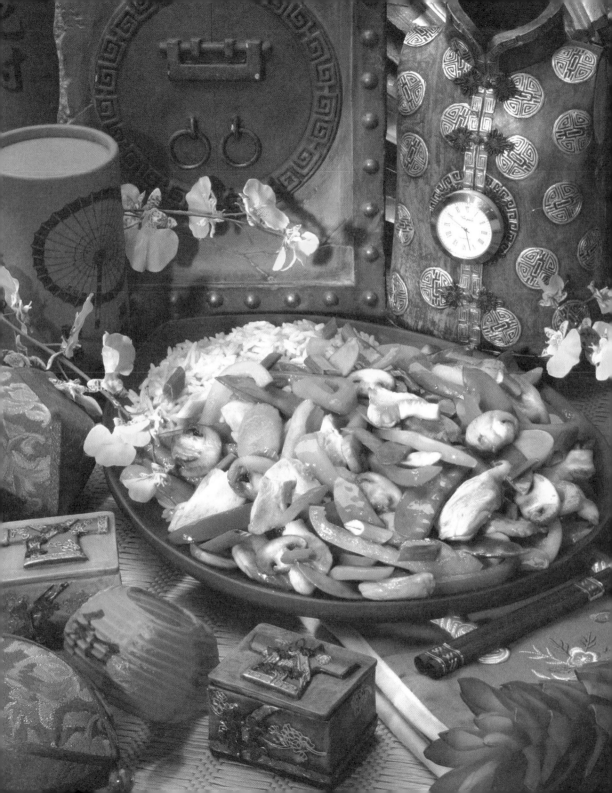

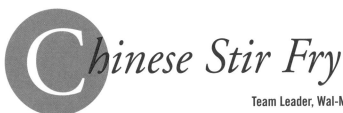

Chinese Stir Fry

Thanks to Scott Berger
Team Leader, Wal-Mart Upper Respiratory, Pfizer

START THE NEW YEAR OFF RIGHT...

...the Chinese New Year that is! It's only minutes to stir fry these colorful ingredients in a *wok*. Consider using the time you'll save to take a *walk* with a friend.

INGREDIENTS

3	boneless, skinless chicken breast halves (approx. 8 oz. each, uncooked)
½ cup	snow pea pods
¼ cup	each, red, yellow and green bell peppers, cut into slices
½ cup	sliced mushrooms
2 tsp.	ginger (1 tsp. if using freshly-grated)
½ cup	low-sodium soy sauce
2 Tbsp.	sugar
½ cup	low-sodium, non-fat chicken broth
	non-fat cooking spray
2 cups	cooked brown rice

PREPARATION

- Brown chicken in non-fat cooking spray, approximately 4 minutes per side or until juices run clear. A wok is best, but a stovetop skillet works fine, also.

- Remove chicken from wok, cut into cubes. Return to wok. Add ½ of the broth and vegetables. Cover and cook 5 minutes.

- Combine remaining broth, ginger, sugar and soy sauce. Pour over chicken and veggies.

- Serve immediately over rice.

NUTRITIONAL ANALYSIS
Servings per recipe: 6
Each serving contains approximately:
335 calories
20 g. protein
56 g. carbohydrates
3 g. fat (1 g. saturated fat)

Fun With Fitness

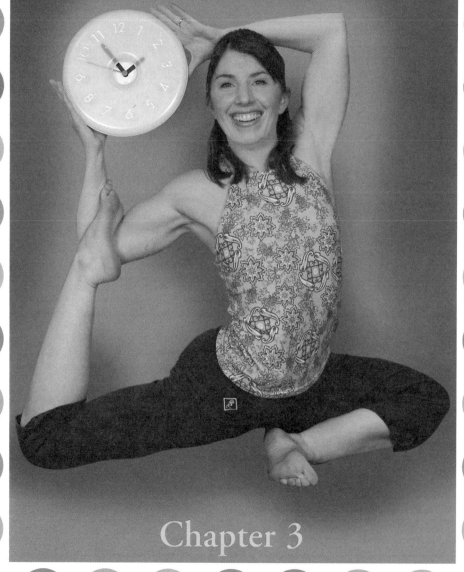

Chapter 3

ROCK AROUND THE CLOCK...

for many fun and active years to come

Many of the greatest joys in life come from physical activity – our ability to get up and go. Think about the joy of lifting your child for a gleeful hug, the joy of strolling hand-in-hand with your sweetheart in the moonlight, or the simple joy of planting bulbs in the garden in anticipation of a bright and colorful spring. The ability to enjoy these activities is part of maintaining a healthy and active lifestyle. Learning to walk, as a baby, is something we all take for granted. Learning to run, as a toddler, is a joy. During those same years, learning to smile and giggle are also treasures. How wonderful if our physical and mental health allowed us to walk, run, smile and giggle as we achieve the wisdom of age. Is it possible? Absolutely... Read on!

The benefits of physical activity go beyond the physical gains of strengthening the heart muscles, improving bone density, boosting energy, lowering cholesterol, improving your immune system, and so on. As we've said, it also includes the all-important psychological effects of self-esteem and confidence, which are boosted by smiles and laughter. What a perfect combination for the right attitude toward exercise. If you put on your smile along with your walking shoes, you'll look forward to exercising and, you'll do it more often... and once you develop a rhythm, you will find it a great stress reliever... and, you'll smile even more! Health experts tell us that laughter is actually a great exercise. In fact, physiologists claim that 15 minutes of belly laughing burns the same amount of calories as 10 minutes of sit-ups. Adopt this attitude, and you'll never again think of exercise as a difficult task. You'll think of it more in terms of activities you enjoy – *like when you were a child and could not wait to go outside and play.*

Healthy lifestyles are about building new habits. You can't make exercise a habit if you are not doing activities that you enjoy. If the treadmill isn't your first choice, try taking your dog for walks in the park or on a local hiking trail. Find aerobics a challenge? Sign up for salsa or country line dancing with a group of friends. Skating or bicycling may be a great alternative to jogging. Just choose something that will make you enjoy the time spent being active.

The key here is to find an activity you enjoy and make it a habit – a healthy habit!

Time Well Spent... Make Exercise Part of Healthy Living

Everyone knows that exercise is good for them, but it still is a matter of choosing to get up and move. If you ask a number of women, some will tell you that they do not have time to exercise because of the demands on their lives. The family, the job, even the pets tend to take priority over what is most important... your health. As Sandra Alridge, a Speaking of Women's Health conference attendee from Houston, Texas, will tell you... "If you don't put yourself first, you may not be there for the kids, the spouse, the job or even the pets." Look for Sandra's story on our Web site at www.speakingofwomenshealth.com.

What better way of showing your family you care for them than by taking care of yourself? You are setting a precedent for them as well as other women in the community. Be a leader and get a group of family and friends together. Walk to improve your health and enjoy the company of others as you walk toward making exercise one of your daily routines.

A sedentary lifestyle is a nationwide problem. According to the U.S. Surgeon General's report, more than 60% of Americans are failing to get the recommended amount of regular physical activity. The key word here is **regular**. It has been reported that 1 out of 4 Americans is not exercising at all, and inactivity among women as they age is much higher than men. **The good news is...** recent research shows that moderate exercise may be as beneficial as intense workouts. Simply put... the adage "no pain, no gain" just doesn't hold true. Walking for 30 minutes a day at an average pace of 17 minutes per mile is beneficial in improving heart-muscle strength and oxygenation. **Even better news...** this same research now shows you can break this into 3 sets of 10-minute walks and you still benefit.

It is common knowledge that inactivity is hazardous to your health and can double your risk of developing heart disease. If you are inactive, you probably tend to eat more. When you eat more and remain inactive, most people will gain weight. This can lead to higher blood pressure, elevated cholesterol and increased risk of diabetes (see Chapter 4 for more information).

The good news is... you can help yourself avoid developing many diseases as you age, if you just start an exercise program and stick with it! Now's the time to get moving!

Walk for Health

Walking has become increasingly popular over the past decade. If you can't run or just don't like jogging, walking can help you achieve many goals, especially cardiovascular health.

A brisk walk will burn the same amount of calories per mile that jogging does (approximately 100 calories). It's important to get your heart pumping during a walk. So gradually include small inclines as you advance in your daily stroll.

Many women find walking a fun alternative to going to a gym. It's something that can be done any time – morning, noon or night. Plus, you don't need to buy expensive equipment to get started. In fact, walking is one of the most inexpensive ways to stay fit and healthy.

During inclement weather, head to your local shopping center, mall or super center for a walk... or, take a class at your local community center.

Start out slowly, and before you know it you'll increase your distance and see great results. Make sure to listen to your body to avoid overexertion and muscle strain. Stretching before and after each walk improves circulation and prevents muscle soreness.

Start the Clock

When beginning an exercise program, use time rather than distance as a measurement. Start with 10 or 20 minutes – whatever is comfortable. If, after 20 minutes you're feeling great... keep going. If not... don't push it. Remember, the key is that you want to get up and do it again tomorrow.

Healthy Benefits of Exercise...

✔ *Strengthens the heart muscle.*

✔ *Enables the body to better use oxygen.*

✔ *Builds energy levels.*

✔ *Lowers blood pressure.*

✔ *Improves muscle tone and strength.*

✔ *Strengthens and builds bones.*

✔ *Helps reduce body fat.*

✔ *Helps reduce stress, tension, anxiety and depression.*

✔ *Boosts immune system.*

✔ *Helps in managing arthritis.*

✔ *Boosts self-image and self-esteem.*

✔ *Improves sleep.*

✔ *Helps you feel more relaxed and rested.*

✔ *Makes you look healthy, fit... even sexy!*

To improve your current physical condition, periodically bump yourself out of your comfort zone. Go a little farther. Go a little faster. After you've picked up your pace, be sure to give yourself plenty of cool-down time. It's all about pace. Avoid the TOOs – **too much, too fast, too soon.**

Learn to ENJOY the act of EXERCISING. Live for the moment. What did you discover, experience or achieve each time you went out? Long-term goals may get you started. But, short-term, achievable goals will keep you moving.

Gear Up for Activity!

✔ A high percentage of people are not wearing the correct size of shoes. We have 26 bones in our feet. Time, weight and gravity cause them to spread out and change.

✔ Typically, our right and left feet are not the same. It is not unusual to have one foot a different size than the other. It is best to be measured and fitted for the longer of the two feet.

✔ Along with the heel/toe measurement, you should also have the heel/ball of your foot measured. You want to try to match up the widest part of your foot with the widest part of the shoe.

✔ When you try on shoes, you are seeking the feeling of overall comfort. Put different styles on each foot at the same time so you can better compare the feeling and fit. The process of being fitted properly is a joint effort between you and the person assisting you. He or she lends their expertise to you while you give feedback as to how the shoe feels.

✔ You want to have the eyelets parallel. A "V" may mean the shoe is too tight. Eyelets bumping together may mean that the shoe is too loose.

✔ The ball of the foot should be comfortably secure in the shoe as you stand or walk around. If it is too loose, your foot will slide around. If it is too tight, your foot is being strangled and irritations will develop.

✔ The foot needs room to expand while you walk or run. There should be a pinch of material across the top of the shoe to allow for this. In addition, you want about a ¼ inch of space in front of the longest toe of the longest foot.

✔ Dress appropriately for the type of activity you engage in. Wear lightweight clothing that breathes and allows sweat to evaporate. Cotton, while comfortable, may not be your best choice because it absorbs perspiration rather than allowing it to move away from the body easily (same goes for socks). Affordable exercise gear can be found almost anywhere. Look for blended fabrics that allow perspiration to "wick away" from the body. The bottom line is, choose sensible, comfortable clothing that does not restrict movement in any way.

Common Exercise Mistakes

It's easy to make mistakes when exercising. All too often, it's because we don't pay attention to proper body form or we push ourself too hard. In either case, these common mistakes may cause problems and derail the goals you have set for yourself.

The most common mistake when exercising is not stretching. You should stretch your muscles before, during and after any physical activity – whether you're running a marathon or simply walking your dog. Proper stretching prevents muscle strains, tearing and soreness. And, don't just stretch your legs…gently roll your neck/head from side to side, reach your arms high overhead, and bend over to stretch all of your back muscles. Think of yourself as a cat waking from a long nap… S-T-R-E-T-C-H!

Another common mistake is not drinking enough water. On a normal day, you should be drinking a minimum of 8 cups (64 oz.) of water. On days that you exercise, you should drink even more than that to rehydrate your body. It's also important to drink water immediately after your exercise and stretching routine to help prevent muscle cramping.

Pace yourself when you work out, and be safe. Remember that even the best athletes didn't happen overnight. It takes PURPOSE, PATIENCE and PERSISTENCE. Enjoy exercise, but do it safely.

Take 4 for Fitness

Stretching or flexibility

Stretching is slow, sustained lengthening of the muscle. Stretching of the arms and legs before and after exercising helps to prevent injury. This is also a great way of increasing range of motion and flexibility. Stretch for 5–10 minutes before and after each exercise routine. It's important to listen to your body as you stretch. Don't overexert yourself. If a certain motion is uncomfortable, then stop. Don't push yourself too hard. In addition to some of the stretching exercises recommended in the paragraph above, there are also stretching exercises that are practices unto themselves... such as Yoga and Pilates. Practicing Yoga and Pilates will also help maintain your flexibility and balance for all of your daily activities.

Strengthening

Strengthening is repeated contractions of a muscle to the point of fatigue. Strengthening exercises make the muscles strong and less likely to fatigue. They also tone the body, improving overall body image. Common strengthening exercises include sit-ups, push-ups, chin-ups and weight-lifting. These resistance types of exercise are wonderful for your bone health. Again, Yoga and Pilates are excellent practices. Can't get to a class? There are plenty of tapes and DVDs available to guide you at home.

Cardiovascular or aerobic conditioning

Cardiovascular activities increase the heart rate for a sustained period of time. They also strengthen the heart and lungs. Swimming, biking and running are common aerobic activities. Studies show that a minimum of 20–30 minutes of aerobic activity 3 times a week is needed to maintain a healthy heart.

Endurance

Another term for endurance is staying power. This is your ability to walk, chase the kids or shop without getting tired. Muscular strength and endurance go hand in hand. They are both necessary to maintain mobility, especially as we age. A resistance type of exercise, such as weight-lifting, improves both muscular strength and endurance.

TIME VERSUS INTENSITY	
Vigorous Activities **More vigorous, less time** **(30–60 minutes 3–4 times a week)**	**Low to Moderate Activities** **Less vigorous, more time (total of** **30 minutes on most days)**
✔ Brisk walking	✔ Washing windows or floors
✔ Jogging	✔ Pleasure walking
✔ Swimming laps	✔ Pushing a stroller
✔ Bicycling	✔ Gardening
✔ Shoveling snow	✔ Housework
✔ Tennis	✔ Dancing
✔ Water aerobics	✔ Golfing
✔ Step aerobics	✔ Yard work

Fire Up Your Metabolism

Your metabolism plays an important role in allowing you to maintain your weight. As we get older, our metabolic rate naturally falls. By increasing your activity, you can "turn up" your furnace and make it work for you.

Here are some ways to "fire up your furnace," according to Ronda Gates, RPh, MS:

✔ Exercise daily, aiming for 10,000 steps a day.

✔ Don't skip meals.

✔ Maintain caloric needs with a lower-in-fat, lower-in-sugar, higher-in-fiber balanced and varied diet.

✔ Do something to improve upper and lower body strength twice a week.

✔ Affirm your intentions several times a day.

✔ Manage stress with laughter, meditation, Yoga and deep-breathing exercises.

✔ Participate in activities that you enjoy.

✔ Do something for someone else – anonymously.

It's *the right time...*

To Read These Fun Tips on Staying Fit

Here are some great tips from Michael J. Hewitt, Ph.D on how to *"Get Fit and Stay Fit to Maintain Your Ideal Weight."*

Go play! Children never look at a clock hoping recess is over so they can get back to spelling or math; rather they're disappointed having to go back inside. However, nearly everyone on the treadmills or stair-climbers is watching the display hoping for the last 5 minutes to pass quickly. That's the difference between "going out to play" and a "workout." Dance, hike, bicycle, ski, kayak, swim... do the thing you love most.

Find an exercise partner. On that morning when you're tempted to hit the snooze button for the third time, but your exercise partner is waiting at the park for your morning walk together, you're going to get up and go. On the day that she's not in the mood for exercise, you are there for her. An exercise partner can be a wonderful motivator.

Cross train. Tri-athletes often have fewer injuries than runners, swimmers or cyclists because they vary their training among three activities and thereby avoid "overuse" injuries common to distance runners or competitive cyclists. Moreover, they become less bored with their training routines because they are different every day. If you exercise in a health club, try spending 10 minutes each on the treadmill, elliptical trainer and the exercise bike, rather than 30 minutes on any one exercise.

Practice balance. If you live long enough, good balance will become even more important than flexibility, strength or cardio-respiratory fitness, because balance helps prevent the fall that fractures the hip. Simple things like dancing, tai chi, boating, not stepping on sidewalk cracks and brushing your teeth while on one foot all stimulate enhanced balance and function.

Subscribe to an exercise magazine or visit the Speaking of Women's Health Web site. Often we fall out of our exercise routine and forget to restart. For a few dollars each month, the publisher will send you a beautiful, four-color, glossy reminder to get back to the activity you love. **Or, for free information, log on to www.speakingofwomenshealth.com and check out our "Health Matters" exercise page.**

Purchase some new exercise clothes. There is something about being dressed appropriately for the ski slopes, for that fitness class or for the bike ride that makes the activity more fun (and usually more comfortable, too). Nothing stimulates you to resume a forgotten activity like having something new to wear for it. Even if you are not perfectly skilled at the activity, you'll look great doing it!

Stretch often, and in small doses. While an hour of Yoga is a superb way to enhance flexibility, a few minutes of gentle stretching daily will be more effective than a full hour of Yoga or a stretch class performed infrequently. Stretching is like showering… a three-minute shower every day is much more effective than an hour-long shower every few weeks!

Leave your exercise equipment out. It is not very inviting to go bicycling if the bike hangs from the hooks in the ceiling of the garage and has a flat tire. Bring it down, fill the tires and lean it against the side of the car. If you have to move it to back the car out of the garage, one day you'll get on it and go for a ride. If you trip over your running shoes every morning while on the way out your front door in your heels, one day you may put them on and go for a walk or run. Keep your exercise clothes in the front of your closet and in the top drawers. If you see them, you'll use them!

Keep an exercise log. You can keep a small notebook tracking your miles walked or your heart rate during aerobics, or you can use the simplest log of all … a wall calendar, a box of gold stars and a goal. The goal should not be to lose 10 pounds or to drop your total cholesterol by 20 points, rather, to exercise so many times during the coming month, and to put a star on the calendar every time you do. You earn a star whether you exercise for five minutes, or for a full hour. If you walk in the morning and bicycle in the afternoon, you earn two stars!

Follow the "five-minute rule." Most people who leave exercise to the late afternoon or evening are too exhausted to start after their busy day. We'll say, "I'll rest today and go twice as long tomorrow." Of course, something comes up tomorrow and exercise is postponed again. When you're too tired for activity, put on your sneakers, go out the front door (or get on the treadmill or exercise bike) and walk around the block so you're back at your front door in five minutes. If after 5 minutes you're still exhausted, stop… your body needs rest more than exercise. Nine times of 10, however, you'll feel better, and the 5 minutes may expand to 10, 20 or even an hour. Even 5 minutes has cardio-respiratory benefits, and even 5 minutes keeps you on your exercise program!

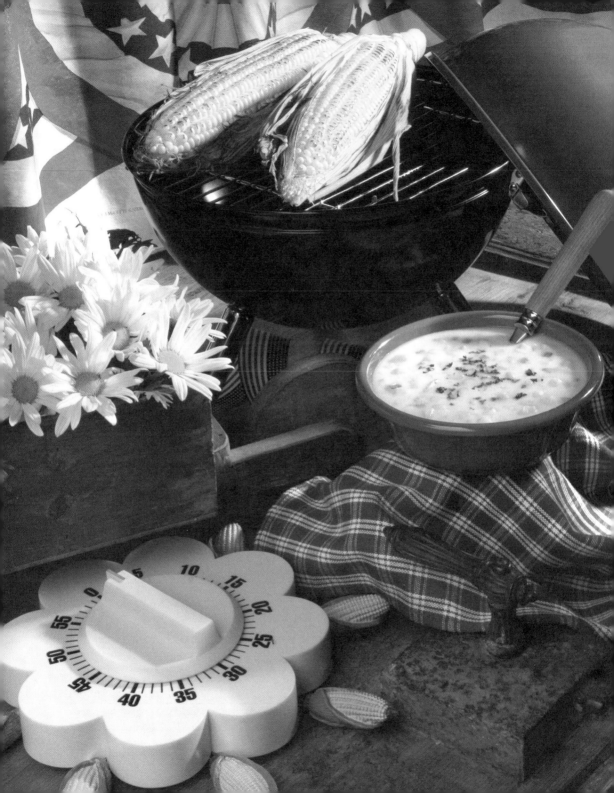

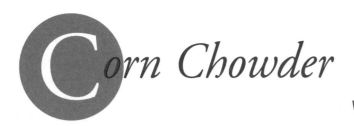

Corn Chowder

Thanks to Ron Schone
Wal-Mart Team Leader, Pfizer

This Fourth of July, serve up this New England classic and you're sure to receive some "oohs" and "ahhs" for your perfect timing. The founding mothers would applaud this low-fat recipe that puts on a spectacular show.

INGREDIENTS

1 Tbsp.	vegetable oil
2 Tbsp.	finely diced celery
2 Tbsp.	finely diced onion
2 Tbsp.	finely diced green pepper
1 pkg. (10 oz.)	frozen whole kernel corn
1 cup	peeled, diced, ½ inch raw potatoes
2 Tbsp.	chopped fresh parsley
1 cup	water
¼ tsp.	salt
	black pepper, to taste
¼ tsp.	paprika
2 Tbsp.	flour
2 cups	non-fat milk

PREPARATION

- Heat oil in medium saucepan.
- Add celery, onion and green pepper and sauté for 2 minutes.
- Add corn, potatoes, water, salt, pepper and paprika. Bring to a boil; reduce heat to medium; and cook, covered, about 10 minutes or until potatoes are tender.
- Place ½ cup milk in a jar with tight fitting lid. Add flour and shake vigorously.
- Add gradually to cooked vegetables and add remaining milk.
- Cook, stirring constantly, until mixture comes to a boil and thickens.
- Serve garnished with chopped fresh parsley.

NUTRITIONAL ANALYSIS
Servings per recipe: 4
Each 1 cup serving contains approximately:

152	calories
6 g.	protein
22 g.	carbohydrates
6 g.	fat (1 g. saturated fat)

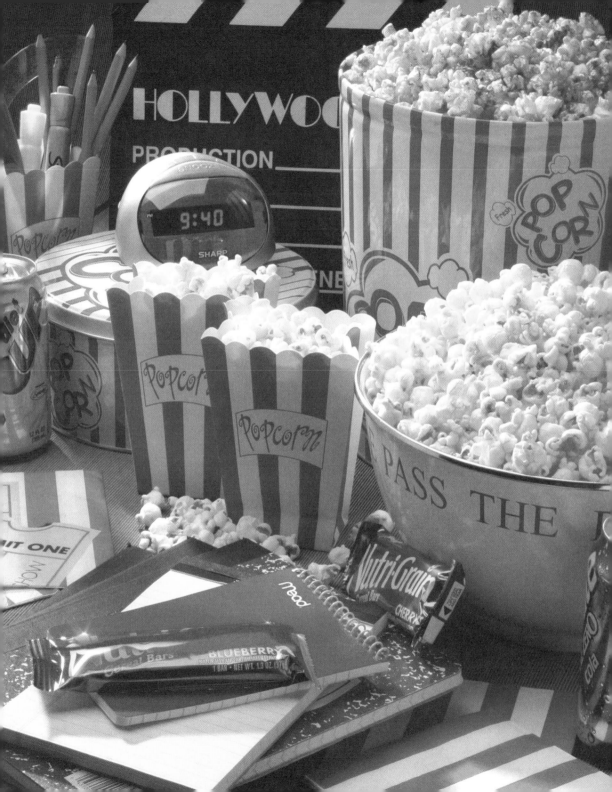

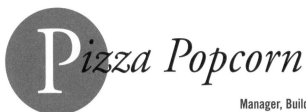

Pizza Popcorn

Thanks to Tina Odom
Manager, Building Brands with Wal-Mart, Unilever

TESTS AND PAPERS GOT YOU BUSY?

Take some time off and invite your friends over for movie night and some pizza… pizza-flavored popcorn, of course! Make it a double feature… see our Web site at www.speakingofwomenshealth.com for a recipe for healthy snack bars to keep you energized during those long study hours.

INGREDIENTS

1 tsp.	dried oregano
1 tsp.	garlic powder
2 Tbsp.	heart-healthy buttery spread
1 bag	microwaveable light popcorn (not butter flavor)
	dash of sweet paprika, for color
3 Tbsp.	grated parmesan cheese, to taste

PREPARATION

- Melt heart-healthy buttery spread and stir in garlic. Pour over popcorn.
- Toss with the oregano, parmesan cheese & paprika.
- Enjoy!

NUTRITIONAL ANALYSIS
Nutritional analysis varies greatly according to brand and formula of popcorn used. Check the label to ensure that "Light" means less than half of the calories come from fat.

Servings per recipe: 2
Each serving contains approximately:

151	calories
2 g.	protein
10 g.	carbohydrates
11 g.	fat

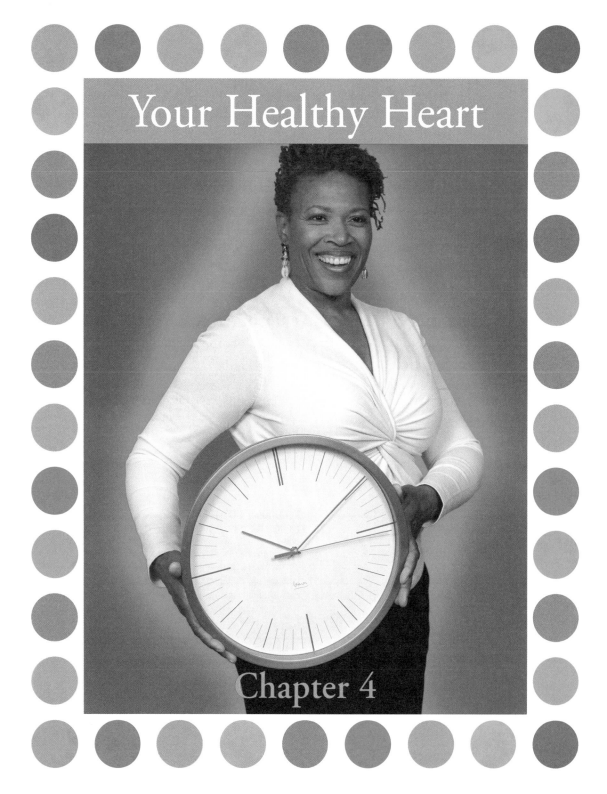

Your Healthy Heart

Chapter 4

YOUR HEALTHY HEART...

Take the time to treasure your ticker

Much like the predictable tick tock of a clock, your heart's beat can be seen as the rhythm of your life. Much like a song, the tempo of your internal ticker tells what you're experiencing – emotionally and, often physically. Just like the music swells as the scene escalates... your heart beat accelerates when you are nervous, "in love" or facing fear. When you relax and are at peace, it slows to a regular, comfortable pace to mark the time of your life. Or, so it should.

Even today, many women think of heart disease as a man's disease. **The truth is...** it is not! Heart disease claims the lives of more than half a million women each year. **The good news is...** with a few simple lifestyle changes, you can significantly reduce your risk factors for heart disease and related diseases, including stroke and peripheral vascular disease.

This chapter will provide information on the different types of cardiovascular diseases, along with the related risk factors. In addition, specific suggestions for reducing your risk factors will be addressed.

The more you know about your risk factors and what you can change, the sooner you can take an active role in your improved heart health. And, more importantly, reduce your risk for heart disease!

Keeping Time

The heart, in its normal healthy state, is a little larger than the size of a closed fist and is a very strong, muscular organ. The heart is the main pumping station for the body. As it contracts, the heart pumps oxygenated blood through the arteries that travel throughout the body. Blood is then returned to the heart through the veins to pick up a new supply of oxygen and start the travel once again.

All muscles need oxygen to work properly. Without the proper supply of oxygen, muscle will die. In the heart, there is a network of medium-sized arteries called coronary arteries that feed the heart muscle. A heart attack occurs when the blood flow in the coronary arteries is diminished. If this occurs, the heart becomes an ineffective pump that may not allow adequate oxygen to reach other parts of the body.

Cardiovascular diseases impact the heart and blood vessel system. Disorders of the circulatory system, such as heart attack and stroke, have killed more women than any other disease process, including cancer, diabetes, lung disease, AIDS, accidents and pneumonia combined. With this staggering fact... the time to learn and understand what you can do to reduce your risk for heart disease is now.

The following pages outline not only the symptoms of a heart attack, stroke and peripheral vascular disease, but the related risk factors as well.

By taking the time to read this chapter and understand your risk factors, you have already taken the first step toward improving your heart health!

Heart Attack

As mentioned, your heart needs oxygen to survive. A heart attack occurs when the blood flow that brings oxygen to the heart is greatly reduced or shut off completely. This happens when the arteries that supply the heart with blood slowly become thicker and harder from a build-up of fat and cholesterol called plaque. A blood clot forms when the plaque breaks free. This clot can block the artery and reduce or shut off the blood flow to the heart muscle. A heart attack, or myocardial infarction (MI), may cause damage or death to a part of the heart muscle. A damaged heart muscle may then cause sudden cardiac arrest (SCA). This is the sudden, abrupt loss of heart function caused by an interruption in the heart's electrical system.

The classic symptoms of a heart attack include chest pain, often radiating down the arm, and mistakenly, many believe that once the symptoms begin, there is no action to be taken until medical help arrives. The fact is, **after calling 9-1-1**, many emergency room physicians recommend taking a full-strength aspirin immediately. Additionally, a heart attack may not always occur quickly, and symptoms may "come and go." For women, the symptoms may be quite different. These include:

✔ A feeling of breathlessness or anxiety

✔ Flu-like symptoms – nausea, clamminess

✔ Pain in the upper back, shoulders, neck or jaw

✔ Unexplained, excessive fatigue and difficulty sleeping

Stroke

Stroke, or "brain attack," is a type of cardiovascular disease that affects the arteries leading to and from within the brain. A stroke occurs when there is blockage of a blood vessel to the brain or a rupture of a vessel wall in the brain. The blockage causes the brain cells supplied by that artery to die because of a lack of oxygen.

Warning Signs of a Stroke:

✔ Weakness in an extremity or loss of sensation – usually one side of the body

✔ Slurred speech, trouble speaking or understanding speech

✔ Double vision or trouble seeing in one or both eyes

✔ Sudden and severe onset of a headache with no known cause

If you or someone with you has any of these warning signs... **Take Action! Dial 9-1-1! Strokes are a serious emergency and need immediate attention. The first 3 hours are the key**. There are clot-busting drugs available that can reduce the long-term disability for most strokes. However, to be effective, they must be administered within 3 hours of the first symptoms.

Peripheral Vascular Disease

This vascular change is usually found in the legs. It also involves the build-up of plaque in the arteries blocking the normal flow of blood to the leg from the heart. When the blood flow becomes limited, the muscles surrounding the artery do not receive the necessary oxygen. This reduction in oxygen causes pain in the hip or leg. If the artery becomes completely blocked, you could develop skin ulcers or even possibly lose part of the limb.

The symptoms of peripheral vascular disease are:

✔ Dull pain in the leg or calf following exercise or walking

✔ Numbness or tingling in the leg or foot

✔ Ulcers or sores on the foot that do not heal properly

✔ A change in skin color

Other changes, such as high blood pressure or kidney disease, have also been noted. All of these symptoms require medical attention and should not be ignored.

Obesity

Obesity is a major risk factor for heart disease and has a direct relationship with diabetes and insulin resistance. Weight loss has shown to decrease the risk for heart disease and increase the production of insulin. In most cases, obesity can be controlled by diet and exercise. If you are 20% over your ideal weight for your height, you are considered to be overweight. Obesity doubles your risk for heart disease. When you lose weight, you may lower your blood pressure and cholesterol, which may then decrease your chance for heart disease. See Chapter 2 for some excellent suggestions for a heart-healthy diet.

It's *the right time...*
To Understand the Risk
Factors of Heart Disease

RISK FACTORS YOU CANNOT CONTROL:

Some women have more risk factors than others relating to cardiovascular disease.

Race – African-Americans tend to have higher blood pressure and therefore are more likely to have heart disease or suffer a stroke.

Family history – Heredity is a risk factor in developing heart disease.

Post-menopausal – There's an increased risk if your ovaries have been removed or you are post-menopausal. After menopause, a woman's risk of heart attack, stroke or peripheral vascular disease is even greater than a man's risk.

RISK FACTORS YOU CAN CONTROL:

There are factors that can contribute to heart disease that can be modified to reduce your risk.

Cigarette smoking – Smoking is the biggest risk factor for heart disease, stroke and peripheral vascular disease.

Weight – Obesity increases your risk of heart disease, stroke and peripheral vascular disease.

High blood pressure – Often referred to as a "silent killer," elevated blood pressure can lead to a heart attack or stroke.

Elevated cholesterol – A 25% reduction in total blood cholesterol can cut the risk of heart disease in half.

Diabetes – Preventing or controlling diabetes reduces your risk for heart disease.

www.speakingofwomenshealth.com

According to recent estimates, nearly 1 in 3 U.S. adults has high blood pressure, but because there are no symptoms, nearly one-third of these people don't know they have it. In fact, many people have high blood pressure for years without knowing it.

Have your blood pressure checked regularly.

Physical Inactivity

Physical inactivity is a major risk factor for both heart disease and diabetes. Proper exercise and weight loss have proven to be an effective way to prevent or delay type 2 diabetes. In addition, exercise and weight management will help keep your blood pressure at healthy levels and reduce the risk for heart disease, stroke and peripheral vascular disease. If you are physically inactive, start an exercise program today! See Chapter 3 for some great exercise tips.

High Blood Pressure

High blood pressure is thought to be the strongest risk factor for heart disease, stroke and peripheral vascular disease. It also contributes to a person being at risk for developing diabetes. The risk for heart disease increases even more when a person has both diabetes and high blood pressure. Know your numbers! The chart below outlines the different classifications for blood pressure.

BLOOD PRESSURE CLASSIFICATION	SYSTOLIC BLOOD PRESSURE	AND	DIASTOLIC BLOOD PRESSURE
Normal	less than 120	or	less than 80
Prehypertension	120-139	or	80-89
Stage 1 Hypertension	140-159	or	90-99
Stage 2 Hypertension	greater than or equal to 160	or	greater than or equal to 100

Source: American Heart Association

Elevated Cholesterol

As your cholesterol level rises, so does your risk for developing diabetes, heart disease, stroke and peripheral vascular disease. The reason for concern is that a high cholesterol level leads to the build-up of fat on the interior walls of the arteries. This build-up can reduce or block the flow of blood, increasing the risk for a heart attack or stroke. Diabetics typically have high triglyceride levels, high levels of LDL cholesterol (bad cholesterol – think "L" for Lousy) and low levels of HDL cholesterol (good cholesterol – think "H" for Happy). The key point is the lower your LDL cholesterol, the lower your risk. A diet low in saturated fat, regular exercise and maintaining a proper weight will all play a major role in keeping your LDL total in an acceptable range. The information below outlines the recommended total cholesterol levels.

Desirable – less than 200 mg/dL

Borderline High Risk – 200–239 mg/dL

High Risk – more than 240 mg/dL

Depending on your personal risk factors, your appropriate level may be different. Consult with your health care provider to determine your ideal LDL/HDL ratio.

Diabetes

Diabetes significantly increases the risk for heart disease, stroke and peripheral vascular disease. As we said in Chapter 2, our bodies convert the majority of the food we consume into glucose, or sugar, to use for energy. The pancreas produces a hormone called insulin that helps the glucose do its job. Diabetes occurs when the body does not produce enough insulin, which causes the sugar level to be too high.

Take Heart!

Most people with diabetes have health problems, or risk factors, such as high blood pressure and cholesterol that increase their risk for heart disease and stroke. When combined with diabetes, these risk factors add up to big trouble. Compared to women without diabetes, women with diabetes have from 2–6 times the risk of heart disease and heart attack and are at much greater risk of having a stroke. People with diabetes often have high blood pressure and high cholesterol and are overweight, increasing their risk even more. In fact, more than 65% of people with diabetes die from heart disease or stroke.

The good news is... many of the same lifestyle choices that help prevent or manage diabetes may also help manage blood pressure, cholesterol and help reduce your risk of heart disease. These include a balanced diet low in fat and rich in fruits and vegetables, moderate daily activity, controlling your weight and maintaining a relationship with your health care team to be aware of your progress.

As many as 50% of people with diabetes are unaware that they have the disease. For this reason, it is particularly important to pay attention to the signs and symptoms of diabetes and its risk factors.

Some of the signs of diabetes are:

✔ Feeling thirsty often

✔ Frequent urination

✔ Feeling very hungry or tired

✔ Weight loss or gain, without trying

✔ Sores that heal slowly

✔ Dry, itchy skin

✔ Tingling or loss of feeling in your feet

✔ Blurred vision

If you are regularly having any of these signs and symptoms, you should tell your doctor.

Diagnosis

The amount of glucose in your blood varies depending on when and what you eat. In general, blood sugar is highest after eating and lowest after you have not eaten for 8–10 hours (usually just after waking). After fasting all night, most people have blood glucose levels between 70 and 100 milligrams of glucose per deciliter of blood (mg/dL). After eating a large meal, a person's blood sugar will rise, but generally not above 140 mg/dL. People with untreated diabetes will have higher blood sugar levels after fasting and after eating.

To determine if you have diabetes, your doctor will test your blood sugar levels. The results of these tests and other clinical findings will be used to decide if you have diabetes and what type. Doctors cannot diagnose diabetes on the basis of one single test. Instead, they will perform two or more glucose tests before confirming your diagnosis. The most common tests to measure glucose are the fasting plasma glucose test, the random blood sugar test and the oral glucose tolerance test.

Before people develop diabetes, they almost always have "pre-diabetes" – blood glucose levels that are higher than normal, but not yet high enough to be diagnosed as diabetes.

	FASTING	AFTER EATING
Normal	70 – 100 mg/dL	below 140
Pre-Diabetes	100 – 126 mg/dL	140 – 200
Diabetes	126 +	200 +

Source: *American Diabetes Association*

There are 41 million people in the United States, ages 40 to 74, who have pre-diabetes. Recent research has shown that some long-term damage to the body, especially the heart and circulatory system, may already be occurring during pre-diabetes.

The good news is... that same research has also shown that if you take action to manage your blood glucose when you have pre-diabetes, you can delay or prevent diabetes from ever developing.

Do the 2-Step

Managing pre-diabetes requires lifestyle changes, namely eating healthier and increasing your physical activity. According to Lisa Porter, M.D., endocrinologist and Director of Clinical Development for Amylin Pharmaceuticals, "It's the combination of diet and exercise that makes a difference... One without the other is not nearly as effective."

What Should You Eat?

If you are overweight or obese, the first step is to lose weight. Studies show that a loss of just 5–10% of your body weight may reduce your risk of developing diabetes by as much as half. Think that sounds like a lot? Consider that if you weigh 200 pounds, 5% is just 10 lbs... that's a good start toward better health. It's important to begin a weight-loss program with the help of your health care team, including, if possible, a dietitian. Together, you can find ways to decrease calories but still consume the foods you enjoy. And, they can suggest strategies to help you change old habits for new ones.

Eating to Control Diabetes

Healthy eating for diabetes includes a wide variety of foods such as vegetables, whole grains, fruits, non-fat dairy products, beans, lean meats, poultry and fish. There is no one "perfect" food, so including a variety of different foods and watching portion sizes is key to a healthy diet. Also, make sure your choices from each food group provide the highest quality nutrients you can find. In other words, pick foods rich in vitamins, minerals and fiber over those that are processed.

Aim for foods that are low in fat and high in fiber. Seek to reduce your portion sizes and eat 5 or 6 smaller meals throughout the day, instead of 3 large meals.

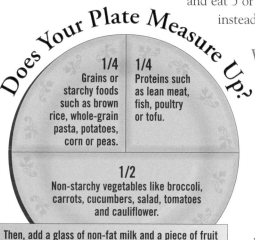

Does Your Plate Measure Up?

1/4
Grains or starchy foods such as brown rice, whole-grain pasta, potatoes, corn or peas.

1/4
Proteins such as lean meat, fish, poultry or tofu.

1/2
Non-starchy vegetables like broccoli, carrots, cucumbers, salad, tomatoes and cauliflower.

Then, add a glass of non-fat milk and a piece of fruit and you are ready to eat!

What About Sugar?

It is widely believed that people with diabetes should not eat any sugar. It would make sense that if the sugar in your blood is too high, you shouldn't eat any more. Well, that's partially correct, but not exactly. Research has shown that sugar has the same effect on blood glucose levels as other carbohydrates, also called carbs, such as bread or potatoes. Calorie-for-calorie, sugar raises blood glucose about the same amount as other carbohydrates. "Modest amounts of sugar are okay, if part of an overall healthy diet," notes Dr. Porter. "Diabetics should avoid any food that raises your blood sugar quickly, or has a high glycemic index."

R$_x$ for Health

Many people with diabetes can manage their disease with lifestyle modifications of improved diet and increased exercise. Over time, a decline in pancreatic function may require additional treatment. **The good news is...** recent advances in medications can have a positive impact. Talk to your doctor or pharmacist.

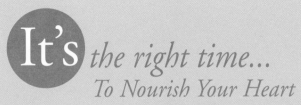

It's *the right time...*
To Nourish Your Heart

Healthy eating is a big part of living a healthy lifestyle. Proper nutrition can increase your overall heart health, as well as help with other diseases, like diabetes and hypertension (high blood pressure).

Everyone wants to eat a diet that will help them maintain a healthy heart and keep veins and arteries plaque-free. But just what does it mean to eat a heart-healthy diet? Recently, the National Cholesterol Education Program provided some new guidelines for a healthy heart. The most important points of these new guidelines are as follows.

NEW GUIDELINES

- ✔ Your diet should include no more than 200 mg of cholesterol daily.
- ✔ Your diet should have no more than 30% of total calories from fat AND most of the fat should be unsaturated.
- ✔ Calories from saturated fat should be limited to 7–10% of total calories.
- ✔ Eat plenty of foods rich in soluble fiber such as oatmeal, beans, peas, fruits and vegetables.
- ✔ Increase physical activity and control weight.
- ✔ If dietary changes, weight control and exercise do not reduce your cholesterol, check with your physician about other options.

A FEW SIMPLE TIPS

A few simple changes in your diet can help to achieve optimal blood fat levels.

- ✔ Switch to very low-fat or fat-free dairy products.
- ✔ Minimize the amount of fat you add to foods. Use more fat-free salad dressings, mayonnaise, sour cream, cream cheese and heart-healthy buttery spreads.
- ✔ Season steamed vegetables with spices and herbs.
- ✔ Bake, broil, grill or boil foods. If you must fry, spray the pan with a non-stick cooking spray or choose a heart-healthy buttery spread.
- ✔ Use liquid vegetable oils rather than solid vegetable shortening. Choose olive, canola or sunflower oils.

Eating a heart-healthy diet and maintaining a good exercise program should be a daily habit to keep your cholesterol down for a long and healthy life. A few healthy choices each day can add up to many years of health and well-being.

www.speakingofwomenshealth.com

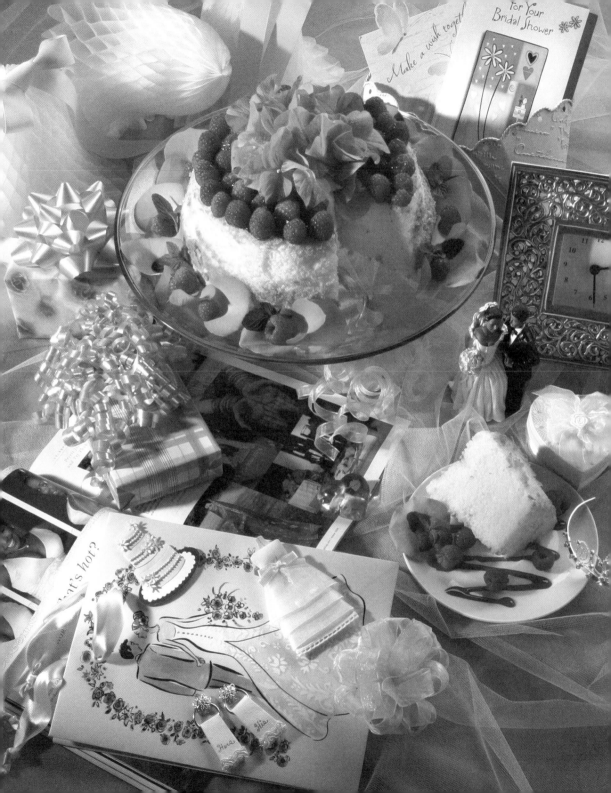

Angel Food Cake *with Raspberry Sauce*

Thanks to Lisa Klauser
VP, Building Brands with Customers, Unilever

Your bridal shower guests will think you're an angel if you serve this cake! Or... bake it tonight and make an ordinary dinner, heavenly!

INGREDIENTS

Cake Batter

1½ cups	egg whites (about 12 eggs)
1 cup	cake flour
1½ cups	plus 2 Tbsp. sugar, divided
1½ tsp.	cream of tartar
1½ tsp.	vanilla extract
½ tsp.	lemon extract
¼ tsp.	salt

Raspberry Sauce

1 cup	raspberries, fresh or frozen
	juice from ½ lemon
4 Tbsp.	no-sugar sweetener, granular

NUTRITIONAL ANALYSIS
Servings per recipe: 16
Each serving contains approximately:

237 calories
2 g. protein
51 g. carbohydrates
2 g. fat

CAKE PREPARATION

- Preheat oven to 375 degrees. Place egg whites in a large mixing bowl and let stand at room temperature for 30 minutes. Sift cake flour and ¾ cup plus 2 Tbsp. sugar together twice; set aside. Beat egg whites with cream of tartar, extracts and salt on medium speed until soft peaks form. Gradually add remaining sugar, 2 Tbsp. at a time, beating on high until stiff peaks form and sugar is dissolved. Gradually fold in flour mixture, a fourth at a time.

- Gently spoon into an ungreased 10-inch tube pan. Cut through the batter with a knife to remove air pockets. Bake on the lowest rack for 30–35 minutes or until top springs back when lightly touched and cracks feel dry. Immediately invert baking pan; cool completely. Run a knife around sides and center tube of pan. Invert cake onto a serving plate.

SAUCE PREPARATION

- Puree berries in blender with lemon juice. Add sugar 1 Tbsp. at a time, to taste. Strain puree through a fine strainer.

- Spoon sauce onto plate, add cake slice, then spoon additional sauce on top.

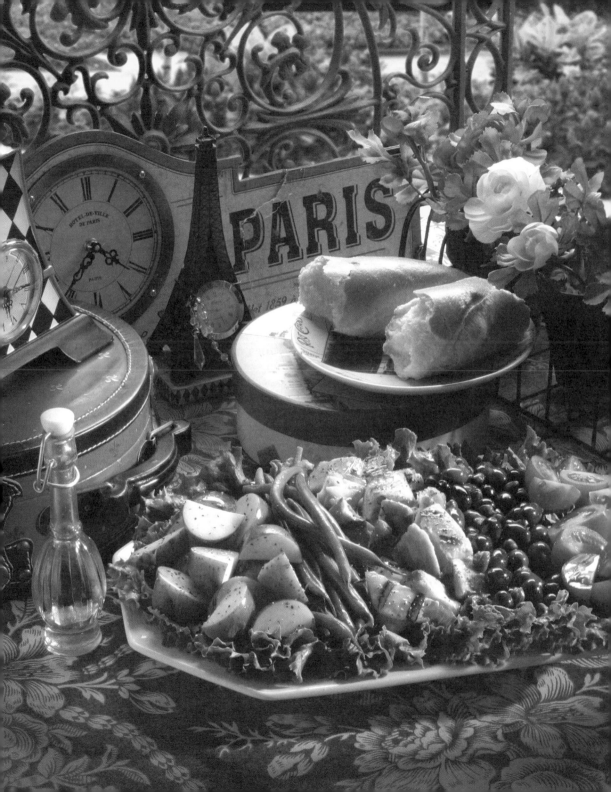

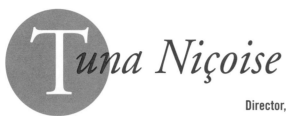

Tuna Niçoise

Thanks to Christine Peddy
Director, Building Brands with Wal-Mart, Unilever

IF YOU LOVE PARIS IN THE SPRINGTIME...

You'll love packing up and going... to a park closer to home, with our picnic of Tuna Niçoise. Put the potatoes, beans, tuna, olives, tomatoes and lettuce in airtight containers. It's only minutes to assemble this one-dish buffet. And, in no time, your picnickers will be dishing up some delicious French cuisine.

INGREDIENTS

1 lb.	tuna steak, grilled
1 cup	fresh greens
1 cup	cherry or grape tomatoes
5	medium-sized new potatoes, cut into quarters
¼ cup	ripe olives
1 cup	fresh, French-style green beans (haricots verts)

Salad dressing (serves 6)

¼ cup	olive oil
2 Tbsp.	lemon juice
	Kosher salt and freshly ground pepper, to taste

PREPARATION

- Grill tuna steak over medium heat approximately 4 minutes per side, until steak begins to flake.
- Parboil or microwave green beans.
- Arrange all ingredients atop fresh greens.
- Sprinkle with dressing and serve immediately.

NUTRITIONAL ANALYSIS
Servings per recipe: 4
Each serving, with 3 Tbsp. dressing, contains approximately:
- 389 calories
- 36 g. protein
- 29 g. carbohydrates
- 15 g. fat (2 g. saturated fat)

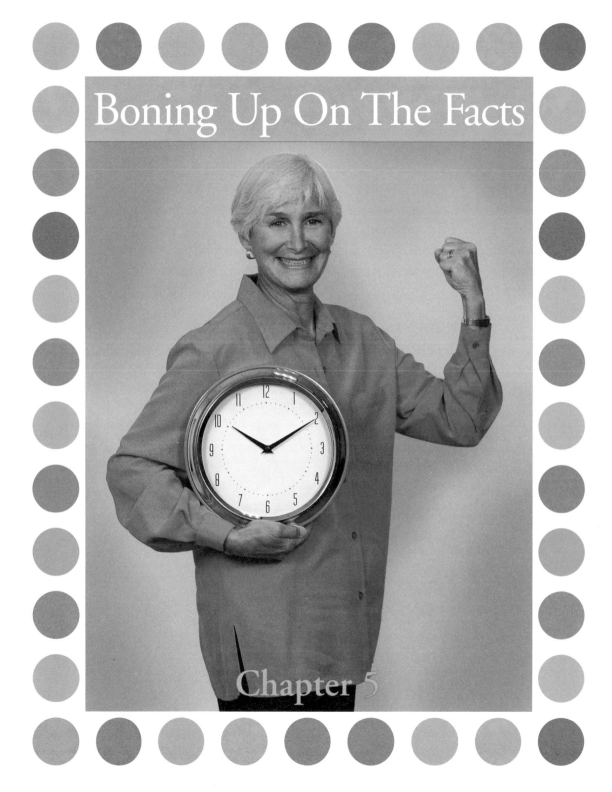

Boning Up On The Facts

Chapter 5

BONE HEALTH...

It's time to "bone up" on the facts

Nature's time for the production of bones is in the first 25 years of life. And, there are lots of ways to encourage young women to ensure that they maximize their body's potential for developing strong bones. Diet and weight-bearing exercise are chief among them. **The great news is...** it's never too late to build strong bones and decrease your risk for bone loss and to prevent fractures... and, we mean at any age.

Osteoporosis has been in the news and a general understanding of the importance of better bone health has become a goal for women's health and well-being. This chapter is to encourage and educate you on how to take your bone health from "knowing about it" to "choosing to do something about it."

Start the Clock for Healthy Bones

The really good news is... it is never too late to improve your bone health. The fact of the matter remains that the critical years for building bone mass begin as a young girl. Some experts believe that through educational programs and continued support regarding the importance of building strong bones early on, a young woman could potentially increase her bone mass by 20%! This is an important factor in protecting you from osteoporosis as you age.

As you grow from a newborn through the age of 25, your bone is steadily renewing and replacing itself to stay dense and strong. As you approach your mid 30s, the ability of the 206 bones in your body to continue construction of new bone to replace old bone gradually diminishes. As part of the natural aging process, your bones begin to break down faster than new bone can be formed. This effect, over time, causes your bones to become thinner, and the holes of the "spongy" inner bone to become larger and weaker. The more fragile your bones, the more likely you are to sustain a fracture. Think a broken bone is no big deal? Think again! According to Lana Holstein, M.D., more women will die from the complications of osteoporosis than will die from breast, uterine and ovarian cancers combined. A great many of these potentially-fatal complications result from an osteoporosis-related hip fracture. Hip fractures may cause immobility. Immobility may result in pneumonia, or a blood clot to the lung, heart or brain. This certainly makes preventing that first fracture "time sensitive,"... doesn't it?

It is important to understand that your framework of bone is not just a hard, lifeless foundation. It is a complex living tissue made of calcium and protein that is constantly remodeling.

By age 25, the average woman has acquired 98% of her skeletal mass. Building strong bones during childhood and adolescence can be the best defense against developing osteoporosis later.

Is Your Framework Collapsing Under Stress?

When bone mass is reduced to a point that the risk of fracture is increased, the condition is called osteoporosis, or porous bone disease. In one's youth, bones could manage through the normal stresses that were brought on every day. Jumping, running, playing and standing were easily tolerated. In someone who has developed osteoporosis, it could be one of these simple actions that may cause a bone to fracture.

It is important to know that not all parts of the skeleton are affected equally. The vertebrae (back bone), jaw and the area near the end of the bones (growth plates... i.e., wrist and ankle) lose bone tissue faster. That is why the hips, limbs, vertebrae and even teeth are more prone to breaks.

The reason why osteoporosis is referred to as the "silent epidemic" is because most women are not aware they have it until a sudden strain, bump or fall causes a fracture. Also, the spine or vertebral column can collapse on itself. Collapsed vertebrae might initially be felt or seen in the form of severe back pain, loss of height or stooped posture called "dowager's hump."

Using Your Time Wisely

The design for healthy bones starts by getting adequate calcium and Vitamin D. They are both important factors in reducing your risk of osteoporosis. The amounts that you need to stay healthy change over your lifetime. The body's demand for calcium is greatest during childhood and adolescence, when your framework (skeleton) is growing rapidly. There is also a great demand for calcium during the child-bearing years and during breastfeeding.

It's never too late to rewind the clock...
you can always "Spring Forward." Here's why it's important to keep your bones strong by renewing their growth.

Your bones provide:

✔ *Structural support for muscles.*

✔ *Protection for your vital organs.*

✔ *Calcium storage essential for bone density and strength.*

Doctors have long recognized the important role Vitamin D plays in helping our bodies absorb calcium, but new research suggests it may be valuable for other areas, including the prevention of certain cancers. The newest research suggests that Vitamin D plays a role in protecting our bodies against lymphoma and cancers of the prostate, lungs and the skin. The strongest evidence is for colon cancer. Since it is nearly impossible to get adequate Vitamin D from food, a supplement may be your best option. And... strive for 10-15 minutes each day of sunshine.

Peri-menopause and menopause are also times when vigilance is necessary. As the body ages, it becomes less efficient at absorbing calcium, due to decreasing estrogen levels. The bones also release calcium faster with the onset of menopause. Remember what we said in the beginning of this chapter... it's never too late to build bone mass and prevent fractures.

Building and maintaining strong bones calls for a healthy lifestyle, including diet and exercise.

Calcium-Rich Diet

In addition to a balance of nutritious, delicious foods necessary for a healthy diet (see Chapter 2), it's also important to concentrate on calcium and Vitamin D. Calcium is a mineral found in many foods. It's not made naturally by the human body. Calcium is important because it is one of the "building materials" needed to maintain healthy bones. Calcium alone cannot prevent or cure osteoporosis, but it's an essential part of the overall prevention and treatment program. While it is very important to get as much calcium as possible from your diet, according to most physicians and nutritionists, it's unlikely that you will reach your daily requirement through diet alone. You may wish to talk to your pharmacist or health care provider about adding a daily supplement of calcium to your diet. The chart on the following page will give you some excellent ideas for foods rich in calcium.

You will see that a rich source of calcium is dairy. However, women who are lactose-intolerant, meaning they cannot tolerate dairy products, have options. There are now commercial preparations of lactose-free foods including milk and dairy products (see the chart on the following page for recommended daily amounts of calcium).

It's *the right time...*
To Stand Up for Strong Bones

Healthy eating habits are important. Eating a balanced diet, rich in calcium, is important. Opt for foods high in antioxidants. Brightly-colored fruits and dark green, leafy vegetables are always a good bet for improved health. Low-fat dairy products such as milk, yogurt, cheese and ice cream are the best sources of calcium. Women need 4 servings of dairy each day to meet the daily requirements.

Other foods that are rich in calcium:

- Orange juice
- Navy beans
- Tofu
- Cereals and breads fortified with calcium
- Sardines
- Turnips
- Almonds
- Kale, spinach and other leafy green vegetables
- Salmon (with bones)
- Broccoli
- Cottage cheese (1% fat)

Soy – The plant estrogens found in soy may help maintain bone density and reduce the risk of fractures, especially in the first 10 years after menopause.

As it was mentioned earlier in this chapter, the recommended daily amounts of calcium and Vitamin D change over your lifetime.

CALCIUM		VITAMIN D	
Age	Daily Requirements	Age	Daily Requirements
9-18	1300 mg	19-50	200 IU
19-50	1000 mg	51-70	400 IU
51 or older	1200 mg	71 and older	600 IU

The U.S. Food & Drug Administration recently reviewed goals for the daily intake of Vitamin D. Called AI (Adequate Intake), the figures supplant the old RDA (Recommended Daily Allowance) and represent the amount of daily Vitamin D in the above age groups.

Source: U.S. Food & Drug Administration

It's Time to Understand New Research on Vitamin D

Vitamin D can be looked at as the "key that unlocks the door" for calcium to be absorbed in the body. Vitamin D helps your body break down and absorb calcium for its full benefit. The exposure of skin to sunlight helps with the production of Vitamin D naturally. Fortified milk also contains Vitamin D. According to Michael Roizen, M.D., of the Cleveland Clinic Foundation, Vitamin D is essential for bone health. (Researchers have also found that getting the adequate amount of Vitamin D may decrease your risk of developing cancer and heart disease substantially.) See the chart on page 67 for your recommended daily intake of Vitamin D.

Exercise... Set Your Clock for 30 Minutes a Day

Exercise is important and will benefit your bones no matter when you start, but you will gain the most benefits if you start young and continue throughout your life. **The good news is...** one of the best exercises for maintaining bone mass is WALKING! All it requires is a good pair of walking shoes and perhaps a friend! It is inexpensive and fun. As your feet hit the pavement, it pulls on the muscles and that helps to maintain bone density. Do this for at least 30–60 minutes, at least 3 times a week. The key here is that walking is weight-bearing, because you are bearing the entire weight of your body.

If you are looking to increase bone density, use strength-training along with weight-bearing exercise. Strength-training helps to strengthen the muscles and bones in your arms and upper spine, while weight-bearing exercises mainly affect the bones in your legs, hips and lower spine.

Got a Minute for Strong Bones?

These exercises help to make your muscles work against gravity. Be careful to avoid exercises that put pressure on your spine.

Cardiovascular workouts. Swimming, elliptical training and cycling are great cardiovascular workouts. However, they are not considered as helpful in improving bone health as are weight-bearing exercises. In each case the water, the machine or the bicycle is bearing your weight.

Build your balance. According to Dr. Hewitt, maintaining your muscle strength will prevent sarcopenia (loss of muscle) and will promote good balance. Balance is as important as bone strength, because it will help prevent falls, which may also help prevent fractures.

Prevent exercise injuries. Warm up before exercising, always stretch properly and vary muscle groups. See an exercise professional for guidance.

A Timely Question… How Do I Know If I Have Osteoporosis?

As we've said, osteoporosis has been called the silent epidemic. A DEXA scan is the gold standard for detecting osteoporosis. This is a state-of-the-art radiology procedure that can determine **bone mineral density** (BMD) or your bone mass. It is a simple, painless procedure that takes 15 minutes and only delivers one-tenth of the radiation of a regular x-ray. The information provided by the test is reviewed by a radiologist and is a useful tool in diagnosing this disease process, particularly in the early stages before broken bones occur. Talk to your health care provider about the right time to have your first DEXA scan.

These measurements from the test can help determine bone strength and the bones that have a potential for breaking. The measurements are reported as T Scores.

UNDERSTANDING YOUR T SCORE		
High Risk	**Medium Risk**	**Low Risk**
Indicates osteoporosis T Score of -2.5 or worse	Indicates low bone mass (osteopenia). T Score of -1.0 to -2.5	Indicates normal bone mass T Score of -1.0 or better

Source: National Osteoporosis Foundation

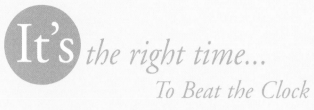

It's *the right time...*
To Beat the Clock

Are you at risk for developing osteoporosis?

There are several risk factors associated with the development of osteoporosis that are common among many women. It's somewhat difficult to predict exactly which women will ultimately develop osteoporosis. Basically, all women are at risk because it can occur in any of us, even without risk factors. However, certain women are at a greater risk than others to develop the disease.

Gender – Women have less bone tissue than do men and lose bone more rapidly because of the changes that occur during menopause.

Age – The older you are, the greater your risk. Bones become weaker and more brittle as you age.

Race – Women of Caucasian and Asian descent are at higher risk. African-American and Hispanic women are at lower risk, but may develop the disease as well.

Family history – A woman's susceptibility to fractures may be in part due to heredity. Women whose mothers or grandmothers have had fractures are likely to have reduced bone mass and have a greater tendency to develop osteoporosis.

Bone structure and body weight – Small-boned and thin women are at greater risk.

Menopause – Women who go through early menopause (either naturally or through surgical removal of the ovaries) are at higher risk.

Lifestyle – Smoking, drinking too much alcohol, consuming excessive amounts of caffeine, and getting too little weight-bearing exercise are all considered risk factors.

Medications and disease – Osteoporosis is associated with certain medications (such as corticosteroids). It is also a recognized complication of certain disease processes, including endocrine disorders, rheumatoid arthritis, certain cancers and immobilization.

Time to Take Action

If you are diagnosed with osteoporosis, there is a range of treatment options. Along with lifestyle changes, there may be medications that will be a part of your course of therapy. The following drugs are approved for the treatment or prevention of osteoporosis:

Bisphosphonates (Actonel®, Fosamax®, Boniva®) – These are oral agents that bind to the bone's surface and block the cells that weaken bone. They are found to be beneficial in reducing fractures. Actonel® and Fosamax® are taken weekly and Boniva® once a month.

Calcitonin (Miacalcin®) – This is a naturally-occurring hormone involved in calcium regulation and bone metabolism. It can be injected or used as a nasal spray. It has been shown to slow bone loss and increase spinal bone density.

Selective Estrogen Receptor Modulators (SERMs) (Evista®) – A "designer hormone" that acts as a weak estrogen to provide benefits of therapy without estrogen risks.

Anabolic Therapy (Forteo®, Teriparatide - parathyroid hormone therapy) – These stimulate new bone formation in the bone remodeling cycle and increase bone density. This is prescribed for men and post-menopausal women and administered as a daily injection.

Estrogen/Hormone Replacement Therapy (Estrace®, Premarin®, Prempro® and many others) – Although FDA-approved, they are no longer considered a first-choice option for prevention of osteoporosis.

No Time Like the Present

You are never too old or too young to improve your bone health. Osteoporosis is not an inevitable consequence of aging. Preventing it should be a health priority for everyone. Although there are some risk factors that can not be eliminated, there are many in your control. How you choose to live your life with healthy eating and exercise reflects in your appearance, attitude and overall well-being.

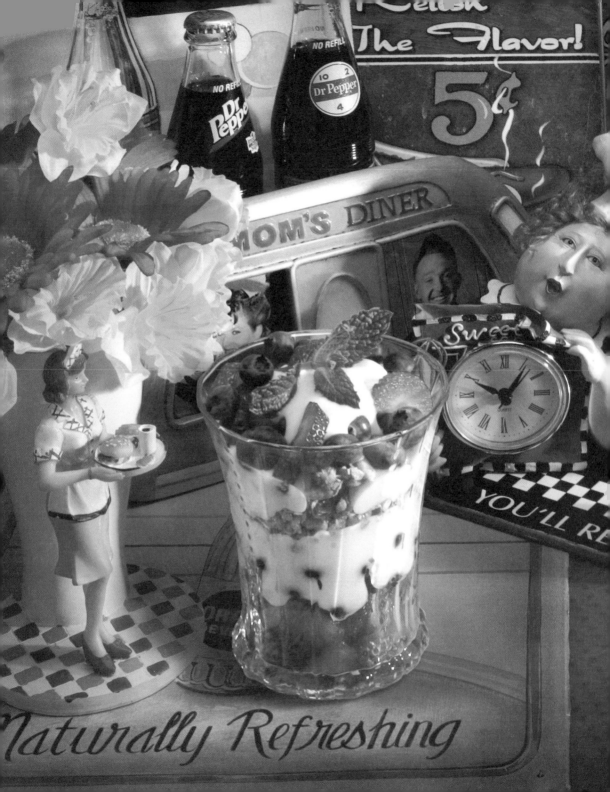

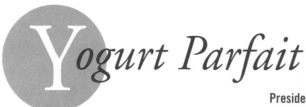

Yogurt Parfait

Thanks to Carol Hamilton
President & General Manager, L'Oreal Paris

Why head to the soda shoppe when you can make your own tasty treat at home?! Rock around the clock tonight with this healthy parfait dessert!

INGREDIENTS

1 cup	vanilla-flavored low-fat yogurt (you may prefer to try another flavor... lemon, peach, berry)
¼ cup	low-fat granola or your favorite cereal
¼ cup	berries (blueberries, raspberries, strawberries, blackberries... or try mango chunks, banana, just about any fruit or berry will do!)

The nutritional value of this recipe can vary greatly depending on the brand and flavor of the yogurt and the type and brand of granola you choose. Be sure to read the labels to ensure you're choosing reduced-fat or non-fat brands of yogurt, and low-fat granola. Log on to www.speakingofwomenshealth.com for a healthy make-your-own granola recipe from Canyon Ranch Health Resorts.

PREPARATION

- Alternate ingredients in a parfait glass beginning with ½ of the yogurt, followed by berries or fruit, and then granola or cereal.

- Insert spoon... Enjoy!

NUTRITIONAL ANALYSIS
Servings per recipe: 1
Each serving contains approximately:

399	calories
17 g.	protein
60 g.	carbohydrates
10.5 g.	fat (3 g. saturated fat)

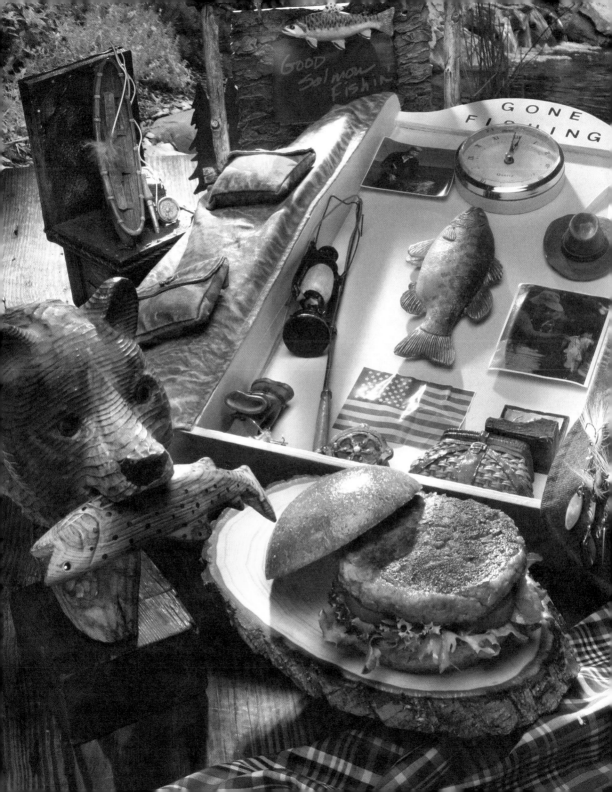

Salmon Burgers

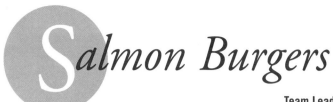

Thanks to Jason Kaiser
Team Leader, Wal-Mart Oral Care, Pfizer

No need to go fishin' for a fresh recipe for a healthy salmon patty. This lunch or dinner dish is a perfect way to catch your heart-healthy Omega-3s. Canned salmon is a staple that's delicious and as good for you as it is easy to prepare. Serve as burgers with lettuce and tomato or serve with a baked potato and green vegetables for a salmon patty dinner.

INGREDIENTS

1 can (15 oz.)	red or pink salmon, packed in water, drained
8	whole-wheat crackers, crushed
¼ cup	seeded & finely-diced red bell pepper
3 Tbsp.	"light" mayo or salad dressing
1 tsp.	lemon juice (bottled or freshly-squeezed)
4 drops	Tabasco sauce
4	whole-grain hamburger buns
4	lettuce leaves
1	tomato (sliced)

Provided with permission from Speaking of Women's Health keynote speaker Zonya Foco, RD, author of "Lickety-Split Meals for Health Conscious People on the Go!"

PREPARATION

- Place drained fish in a medium bowl (remove some of the skin, if desired); flake fish with a fork, mashing bones (great calcium).
- Add the next 5 ingredients and mix well.
- Shape the salmon mix into 4 patties.
- Coat a large nonstick skillet with cooking spray and place over medium heat; cook salmon cakes, turning once, until lightly browned on each side.
- Assemble into burgers.
- Serve with vegetables.

NUTRITIONAL ANALYSIS
Servings per recipe: 4
Each serving (1 salmon burger including the whole-grain bun, contains approximately:

370	calories
26 g.	protein
35 g.	carbohydrates
12 g.	fat

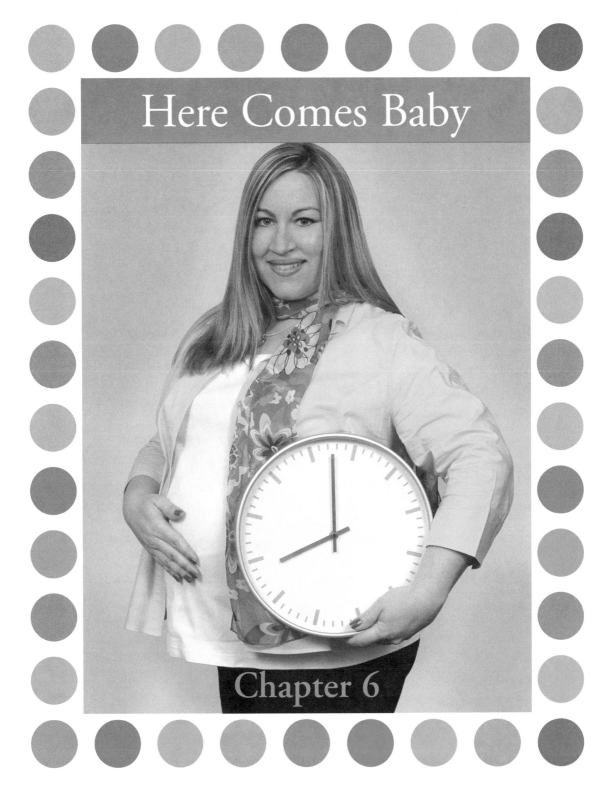

Here Comes Baby

Chapter 6

A MOMENT IN TIME
GREAT EXPECTATIONS...

for a healthy pregnancy.

When baby makes 3 or 4 or 5...

Congratulations...You're Pregnant!

The time is right... and, your body is its own 9-month clock. You've got GREAT EXPECTATIONS... and you've probably got a lot of questions, too. Whether this is your first child or your third, this chapter is designed to help answer those questions. You'll be going through some changes during the following months, both physical and emotional. At times, you may wonder "Is this normal?" This chapter will help you with these issues and keep you informed. Refer to it when you have specific questions. The answers may be right here. For the first few weeks after your pregnancy is confirmed, all you'll be able to think is, "I'm really pregnant." It's a happy and emotional revelation. You may also be thinking about the impact on your life, your family, your budget and other matters. This can be a fun time of learning and planning.

In Due Time

If it's true "you are what you eat"... then certainly what you eat influences your baby's health and well-being. While we once thought that "the baby will take what it needs from the mother," obstetricians and nutritionists now firmly believe that the health of the baby at birth and beyond, as well as the health of the mom, depends greatly upon her nutrition during the pregnancy.

In order to plan for a healthy pregnancy for you and your baby, this chapter is designed to help you better understand what you and your baby need during the next 9 months, and beyond if you plan to breastfeed.

During pregnancy, it's not just important to think of how much you eat... it's equally important to consider what you eat. A pregnant woman needs about 300 calories more each day to stay healthy and nourish her baby. Those extra calories should come from nutritious foods, so they can contribute to your baby's growth and development.

In order to gain weight in a healthy manner, eat a variety of foods each day for breakfast, lunch, dinner and snacks. Experts recommend that you eat 3–5 small meals spread over the day. Make sure that your meals include the number of servings of the basic foods you need each day. Please review the Food Pyramid Guide in Chapter 2. You should be able to increase the Food Group servings overall in order to sensibly gain weight; i.e. instead of 2–4 servings of fruits, increase it to 4 or more servings.

As well as eating properly, make sure that you are getting enough water. Try to drink about 6–8 cups of liquids each day. In addition to water, milk, fruit juices and vegetable juices are ideal. Although this may seem counter-intuitive, water actually helps eliminate fluid retention by flushing your system. And, this should be a healthy habit for life.

According to G. Byron Kallam, M.D., from the Medical Clinic of North Texas, the link between what you eat during pregnancy and the health of your baby is much stronger than once thought. That's why doctors now agree that NO amount of alcohol consumption should be considered safe. If you smoke... STOP immediately! Smoking deprives your baby of needed oxygen, causing him or her to develop and gain weight more slowly in the womb, and has been linked to other serious complications, as well as attention deficit disorder and other behavioral problems. Talk to your doctor or pharmacist for help to stop smoking.

The use of caffeine during pregnancy is controversial, but you won't get any arguments from your obstetrician or midwife if you choose to cut back on your intake. One thing's for sure: You'll feel better if you cut back on caffeine. It's a stimulant, so it increases your heart rate and metabolism and can cause insomnia, nervousness and headaches. It may contribute to heartburn by stimulating the secretion of stomach acid. It's a diuretic, so it makes you urinate more often and become dehydrated more easily. **The good news is...** today there are plenty of "better for you" options from which to choose. Look for caffeine-free sodas, fruit juices, herbal teas or flavored waters. If you must have your morning coffee or latte, choose decaffeinated, or half-caf. Most experts agree that up to 300 mg of caffeine per day will not harm your baby.

A Day of Healthy Eating for Two!

Whether you're pregnant or not, a healthy diet includes proteins, carbohydrates, fats, vitamins, minerals and plenty of water. Food labels will tell you the kinds of nutrients that are in foods, and are listed on the labels with the letters RDA, which stands for Recommended Daily Allowance. This is the amount of a nutrient recommended for daily consumption. When you're pregnant, the RDAs for most nutrients are higher.

Protein is needed for cell growth and blood production. It is found in lean meats, fish, poultry, egg whites, beans, peanut butter and tofu. You need about 70 grams per day, or roughly 10% of your calories (3–4 servings daily, or one with each meal or snack).

Carbohydrates are necessary for daily energy production and should make up about 50% of your caloric intake. Choose complex carbs, which come from whole-grain breads, cereals, brown rice, fruits and vegetables. Simple carbs come from sugars, and contain fewer nutrients for your growing baby.

Fats are needed to help the body store energy, which is essential for baby's growth. The key is to choose good fats, which typically come from meats, dairy products and nuts and seeds. No more than 30% of your daily caloric intake should come from fats, and fewer than 10% of your calories should come from saturated fats.

The Essential 3

During pregnancy, 3 nutrients are more essential than ever – calcium, iron and folic acid.

Calcium builds strong bones and teeth, and assists with muscle and nerve function. Calcium is found in milk, cheese, yogurt, sardines, salmon with bones, spinach and other dark green leafy veggies.

Iron is needed for red blood cell production and is found in lean red meats, spinach, and fortified whole-grain breads and cereals.

Folic acid (folate) helps prevent neural tube defects, including spina bifida. Even before you're pregnant, experts recommend that you increase your intake of folic acid. This development begins in the earliest stages of pregnancy, so most doctors recommend that women planning to become or who are pregnant begin a supplement with folic acid immediately. Food sources of folic acid include green leafy vegetables, dark yellow fruits and beans, peas and nuts. Folic acid is also essential for a healthy heart throughout life.

If you are a vegetarian, it may be difficult to get the added amounts of protein, vitamins and minerals from your diet. Talk to your health care provider about the nutrition you need. Most will recommend a supplement for added calcium, folic acid and Vitamins B12 and D.

Because many pregnant women become constipated from the added iron in their diets and supplements, it's important to increase your intake of fiber to about 30 grams per day. The best sources are fruits, vegetables and whole-grain breads and cereals. This is another reason it is essential that you load up on water and fluids, which will help keep you regular (and comfortable).

Weight Gain

It is generally recommended that a woman of normal weight before pregnancy gain between 25 and 35 pounds during pregnancy. If that sounds scary... consider how it adds up:

7.5 lbs. →	average baby's weight	4 lbs. →	your body's extra fluids
7 lbs. →	your body's extra stored protein, fat and other nutrients	2 lbs. →	breast enlargement
		2 lbs. →	enlargement of your uterus
		2 lbs. →	amniotic fluid
4 lbs. →	your extra blood	1.5 lbs. →	placenta

Most women lose up to 10 pounds during birth alone, and your body quickly adjusts its retained fluids. According to many obstetricians, breastfeeding also helps shrink the uterus back to its normal size quickly.

It's *the right time...*
To Get the Vitamins and Nutrients You Need

Vitamin A – Promotes healthy skin, eyes and growing bones (carrots, dark green leafy veggies and sweet potatoes... think orange and green).

Vitamin C – Supports healthy gums, teeth and bones, and helps with iron consumption, as well as protects tissue from damage (citrus fruits, strawberries, tomatoes, broccoli, dark leafy vegetables and fortified juices).

Vitamin B6 – Helps the body effectively use proteins, fats and carbs (pork, whole grains and bananas).

Vitamin B12 – Needed for nervous system development and red blood cells (beef, fish, poultry, eggs and milk).

Vitamin D – Essential for healthy bones and teeth and aids in the absorption of calcium (fortified milk, dairy products, cereals and breads).

Calcium – Aids in skeletal development (milk, yogurt, cheese, spinach and dried beans).

Folic Acid (Folate) – Helps prevent neural tube defects (green leafy vegetables, dark yellow fruits and beans, peas and nuts).

Iron – Essential for making red blood cells (liver, seafood, wheat germ, whole grains and dark leafy vegetables).

Magnesium – Helps promote healthy nerve and muscle formation (peas, nuts, whole grains and dark leafy vegetables).

Protein – Provides amino acids, which are the building blocks of your baby's body (beef, pork, chicken, eggs, milk, cheese, legumes and nuts).

Zinc – Formation and growth of fetal cells (meat, eggs, seafood, whole grains and dried beans).

Sensible Guidelines for Prenatal Exercises...

Common sense, listening to your body's signals and talking with your health care provider are the main guides to exercising during pregnancy. Normally, you don't have to limit your exercise, except when it risks injury to you or your baby. When exercising, drink lots of water and wear good shoes and a support bra. You should stop any exercise if you develop shortness of breath, chest pain, extreme fatigue, dizziness, uterine contractions, decreased fetal movement or leakage of fluid from the vagina.

Be sure to discuss your exercise routine with your health care provider.

Exercise

Whether you are planning to have a "natural" childbirth with little or no anesthesia, or whether you choose some pain-reducing drugs, you still need to exercise during your entire pregnancy to develop muscle strength for labor. Exercise also helps with backaches, circulation, insomnia and weight control. If you experience certain complications during your pregnancy, you and your baby would probably benefit from a more sedentary activity level with little exercise. If you are expecting twins, have high blood pressure, an incompetent cervix or a condition in which it appears that your fetus is not growing properly, bed rest or little exercise may be recommended.

Certain types of exercise are safer during pregnancy than others. Walking and swimming are two such examples. Aerobic classes, such as water and low-impact aerobics, and those designed especially for pregnancy are beneficial. Other exercises such as running, racquet sports and weight-training should be done in moderation. They are more appropriate for those pregnant women who did them prior to pregnancy.

Here are a few exercises to help prepare your body for labor, and to help keep you active throughout your pregnancy:

The Pelvic Rock – This is probably the most common exercise taught in childbirth classes and for good reason – it is excellent. You can use it before and after delivery, first to give the fetus good support and then to firm those abdominal muscles. You can do the exercise standing or in the "all fours on the ground" position.

Standing Up (The Pelvic Rock) – Keep your back straight, tighten your buttocks, bend your knees slightly, and rock your pelvis back and forth. This is actually a belly dancing technique, called the hinge. To enjoy your daily exercising more, put on some music and slowly walk about doing this exercise. Your abdomen and bottom should work like a hinge, while the rest of your body stays upright. Once you get the hang of it, you can understand why belly dancing is so popular as a form of exercise, even for pregnant women…it is fun!

All Fours (The Pelvic Rock) – Get on your hands and knees with your legs and hands parallel to the floor. Pull your buttocks down and slightly arch your back, tilting your pelvis forward. Then push your buttocks out and back, tilting your pelvis back. Don't let your back curve in as the pelvis is rocked.

Kegel Exercises – You can do this exercise to tone muscles in the pelvic area and improve circulation. Kegels involve controlling and relaxing certain sets of pelvic muscles, one at a time. First, contract your muscles like you are holding back urination. Then, tighten your muscles like you are holding back a bowel movement. Finally, contract the vaginal muscles. It may take some practice to isolate each of these sets of muscles, but keep practicing. Relax and contract each set of muscles separately, contracting them harder and longer each time. This exercise should be continued after delivery to promote more rapid healing and to improve the tone of the vagina.

The Squat – Stand with your back against a wall. Lower your body slowly down the wall, with your hands against it, until you are in a squatting position. Keep your feet parallel and your heels flat against the floor. Then, slowly raise yourself back up. A variation of the squat: hold onto a heavy piece of furniture that won't tip over, squat down, keeping your heels flat on the floor and your back straight, and letting your knees spread open. Slowly rise back up. Practice both types of squat exercises daily.

For more information and to view illustrations of these exercises,
log on to www.speakingofwomenshealth.com

Changing Times

With the exciting news of your pregnancy now a reality, you can expect some changes to occur. The following outlines some of the expected changes along with tips to help manage them. Remember… these changes are normal and just part of the wonderful pregnancy process!

Breasts – From the beginning, your breasts may be larger, firmer and more tender than usual. The areola (the dark area around the nipples) may get larger and grow darker in color. Halfway through your pregnancy, your breasts may start to secrete fluid (colostrum) in small amounts. Be sure to keep them clean with frequent washings, and toward the end of your pregnancy, you may want to put gauze pads inside your bra to protect your clothes.

Morning Sickness...

...it isn't necessarily confined to the morning hours. Few women suffer with nausea after the fourth month, but if it is unusually severe, call your health care provider. You need to keep food down to grow a healthy baby.

Morning Sickness Remedies:

✔ *Eat bread or crackers before you get out of bed each morning.*

✔ *Get out of bed slowly – don't jump up.*

✔ *Try yogurt, milk or juice before bedtime.*

✔ *Avoid greasy, fried foods or spicy, heavily-seasoned foods.*

✔ *Eat several small meals during the day rather than a few large meals.*

✔ *When sick, get fresh air, take deep breaths and sip soda water.*

Urination – When your uterus expands, it may put pressure on your bladder. The need to urinate is common in the first stages of pregnancy, and in the last weeks. Don't try to control this issue by drinking fewer fluids. Your baby needs you to drink at least 8 cups (64 oz.) of liquids a day. If you experience frequent urination that is accompanied by pain, burning and fever, consult your health care professional immediately.

Heartburn – Check with your doctor or pharmacist first, but most agree it isn't your heart that is burning, it's common indigestion! It's all right to use an antacid preparation, but do not use baking soda or sodium bicarbonate preparations for your heartburn. Before you buy an over-the-counter remedy, ask your health care provider which they recommend. In severe cases of heartburn, you might want to have the head of your bed elevated to encourage your stomach fluids to stay put! (Ask someone to add 4″ of books beneath the head posts to elevate the head of the bed temporarily.)

Constipation – Drink lots of fluids to avoid constipation, a common complaint of pregnant women. Exercise every day and eat plenty of fruits and raw vegetables. Try nutritional remedies first, including the addition of bran and bran products to your diet. Don't be shy about discussing this problem, because it is common during pregnancy.

Backache – As your womb grows, your pelvic bone joints relax, which can cause pain in your lower back. Comfortable shoes and good posture may help, but exercise will probably relieve your backache more than anything else. With the help of your health care provider, develop a routine of back exercises every day from the beginning of your pregnancy. See Page 82 for some great prenatal exercises that will help strengthen your back and pelvic muscles.

Insomnia – Many women find it helpful to do some mild stretching and relaxation, such as Yoga and meditation, to help them rest easier. It is important not to take sleeping pills or drink alcohol to try to solve this problem. Physicians and researchers agree that NO amount of alcohol is safe for use during pregnancy.

Varicose Veins – Varicose veins are caused when the veins in your legs get weak and enlarge with blood. They have to work harder to carry blood back up your legs to your heart. Sometimes pregnancy can aggravate this problem. The swelling uterus partially cuts off circulation from your legs. Exercise will help. Don't stand for long periods of time without moving. When you sit, try to prop your legs up to make return circulation easier. Varicose veins are more of a problem for women having their second or third child. But, even if you are having your first baby, try to do as much as you can to aid the circulation in your legs.

Hemorrhoids – Many women suffer with hemorrhoids, or get hemorrhoids for the first time while they are pregnant. Hemorrhoids are enlarged veins right at the opening of the rectum. Though they are sometimes due to the blockage of circulation caused by the increased size of the baby you are carrying, they are also frequently caused by the straining due to constipation. If you do suffer with hemorrhoids, try lying on your side with your hips elevated on a pillow. The key is to prevent hemorrhoids by eating fruits, raw vegetables, bran products and adding water to your diet every day.

Swelling – Pressure from the growing uterus and your changing hormones can cause swelling, especially in your legs. Dr. Kallam cautions to avoid excessive sodium intake, which will only make you retain more water. Brief periods (up to 2 days) of bed rest are usually the best treatment.

Contractions – The uterine muscle contracts spontaneously from early pregnancy until the onset of real labor. Usually the contractions are irregular and painless (Braxton-Hicks contractions) and may produce "false" labor if they become painful. If they become progressively closer together, last longer and become more painful, notify your health care providers so they can make certain you are not in early labor.

Father Time marches on…but Mother Time ROCKS!
Enjoy quiet moments rocking your baby while listening to music. Cherish these
moments… they are soothing to you and your baby, and, according to research,
listening to classical music, even before birth, helps to develop logic
and critical thinking for life.

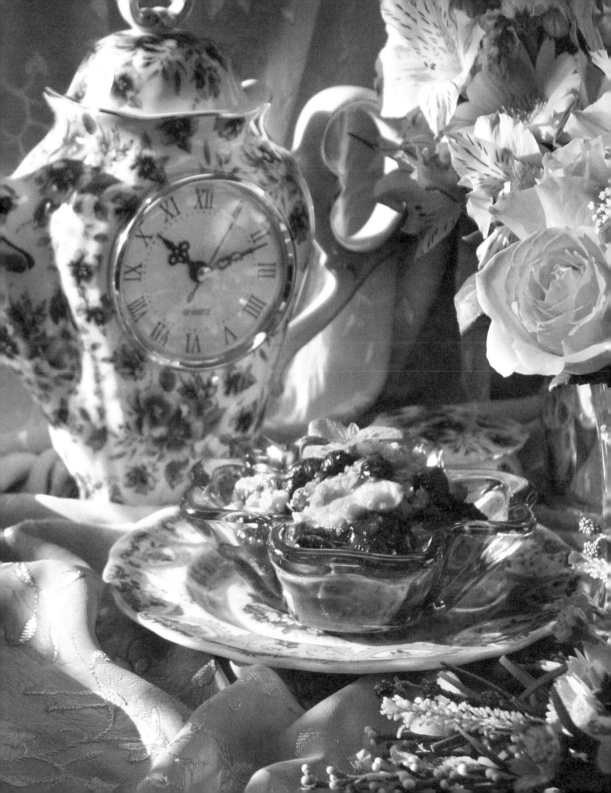

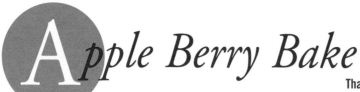

Apple Berry Bake

Thanks to Elaine Plummer
External Relations Manager, Procter & Gamble Pharmaceuticals

TEA TIME

"Tea for two" can easily make room for three or more with this "berry" delicious dessert, chock full of antioxidant-rich fruits!

INGREDIENTS

Filling

4 cups	peeled, thinly-sliced apples (about 4 medium)
2 cups	fresh or frozen blueberries (do not thaw) or sliced strawberries
¼ cup	firmly-packed brown sugar
¼ cup	frozen orange juice concentrate (thawed)
2 Tbsp.	all-purpose flour
1 tsp.	ground cinnamon

Topping

1 cup	quick-cooking oats, uncooked
½ cup	firmly-packed brown sugar
5 Tbsp.	heart-healthy buttery spread, melted
2 Tbsp.	all-purpose flour

PREPARATION

- Preheat oven to 350 degrees. Spray 8-inch square glass baking dish with cooking spray.
- For filling, combine all ingredients in large bowl; mix until apples are evenly coated. Spoon into baking dish.
- For topping, combine all ingredients in small bowl; mix well. Sprinkle evenly over fruit.
- Bake 30–35 minutes or until apples are tender. Serve warm.

NUTRITIONAL ANALYSIS
Servings per recipe: 9
Each serving contains approximately:
  252 calories
  2 g. protein
  50 g. carbohydrates
  6 g. fat (1 g saturated fat)

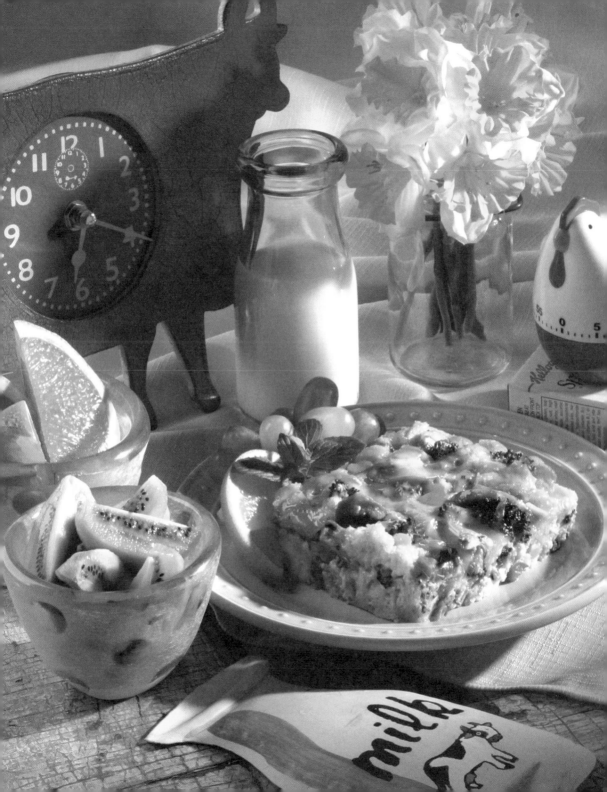

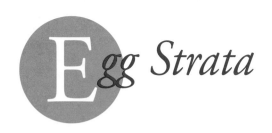

Egg Strata

Thanks to Lori Kumar
Merchandise Manager, Wal-Mart

When the cock crows, the cow moos and the alarm goes off, wake up and set your timer for this "egg-sceptionally" great breakfast.

INGREDIENTS

1 tsp.	olive oil
2 Tbsp.	shallot, peeled and diced
2 cups	variety of vegetables; choose from fresh spinach, broccoli, tomato, onion, mushroom
7	egg whites (if using fresh eggs, whisk egg whites with a fork until slightly frothy; otherwise use prepared egg whites)
1	whole egg
6 oz.	turkey or chicken sausage, skin removed
1 cup	non-fat milk
3 oz.	low-fat cheese, grated
1 tsp.	herbs (oregano, dill, thyme, basil)
	salt and pepper, to taste
2	slices whole-grain bread, cubed

PREPARATION

- Prepare sausage according to package directions. Set aside to cool.
- Sauté shallot in olive oil and herbs for 1 minute. Add vegetables, beginning with onion and broccoli, adding mushrooms, tomatoes or spinach last.
- Meanwhile, whisk together egg whites, egg and milk.
- Process sausage until crumbled in food processor.
- In a glass baking dish coated with cooking spray, cover bottom with bread cubes. Crumble sausage, then add veggies. Pour egg and milk mixture over top. Sprinkle with cheese.
- Cover and refrigerate overnight.
- In morning, uncover and bake at 350 degrees for approximately 45 minutes, or until browned and baked through.

NUTRITIONAL ANALYSIS
Servings per recipe: 6
Each serving contains approximately:

169	calories
17 g.	protein
7 g.	carbohydrates
8 g.	fat (4 g. saturated fat)

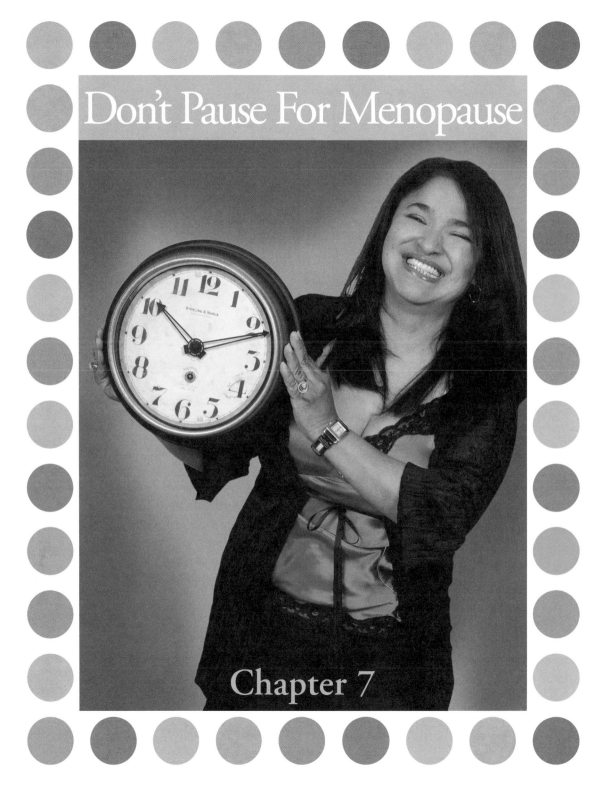

Don't Pause For Menopause

Chapter 7

THE HANDS OF THE CLOCK GO AROUND...

and bring new pleasures to celebrate the "Time of Your Life"

Wouldn't it be great if we all had the wisdom to see how time gives us grace, patience, freedom and, above all...humor?

With a bit of that humor in mind, think about how you watch the clock waiting for your workday to end, and the fun to begin. Think about menopause in the same way! Your reproductive system has been at work for about 40 years... it's now time to have some fun!

As the hands of the clock move around, minute by minute and hour by hour, there is something very reassuring about the consistency of that movement. Only recently have women been taking more control of their own personal health and well-being. It is exciting to see women who are knowledgeable about life's transitions and learning to embrace the changes.

Menopause is a normal phase of a woman's life and should not be looked at as an illness or something that needs to be fixed!

What is premature menopause?

Premature menopause happens before the age of 40 – whether it is natural or induced. Factors include:

✔ *Family history*

✔ *Medical treatments*

✔ *Surgical removal of the ovaries*

✔ *Eating disorders*

✔ *Cancer treatments*

Having premature menopause puts a woman at greater risk for osteoporosis and heart disease later in her life. See the chapters on osteoporosis and heart disease to minimize your risks.

What is Menopause?

Menopause (or "the change" as our mothers and grandmothers called this time of life) is not one singular event. It is a transition that can start in your 30's or 40's and may last into your 50's or 60's. The actual definition of menopause is when you have not had a menstrual period for one full year. The average age for women to enter into menopause is 51. Many women will start to experience signs and symptoms well before their periods actually end.

Women are born with close to 1 million eggs. Through the aging process, the ovaries slowly shut down hormone production. In the past, researchers and physicians looked at menopause as the ending chapter of a woman's life.

Luckily, we now know that menopause is not the beginning of the end, but the beginning of a new chapter in our lives. We should look upon this time with a new sense of freedom, excitement and energy.

Peri-Menopause

Peri-menopause, or menopause transition, is the time during which a woman's body starts to make less estrogen and progesterone, and she starts to experience menopausal signs and symptoms. **The good news is...** not all women have symptoms. In fact, fewer than 2% of women have symptoms severe enough to interfere with daily activities. Peri-menopause can last anywhere from 2–10 years. As with pregnancy, there are no 2 women who will exhibit their transition the exact same way. For example, one woman may have night sweats that wake her frequently. Another woman of the exact same age may not even be aware of the change at all. The more that is learned and understood about the changes, the more positive transition we will have as women. To fully understand this phase of a woman's life, it is best to be aware of the common signs and symptoms that have been reported.

Here is a list of symptoms that you may experience during peri-menopause.

Irregular Periods: Irregular periods are what most women experience first. How much you bleed may change. It could be lighter or heavier. Periods may be shorter or last longer. These changes are normal and are caused by changes in the reproductive system.

Here are some reasons for concern. Talk to your health care provider if:

✔ Your periods are coming very close together

✔ You are bleeding heavily or have clots

✔ You spot constantly

✔ Your periods are lasting more than one week

Hot Flashes: Another common symptom reported among women is hot flashes. As our Speaking of Women's Health humorist and speaker Suzanne Metzger says, she prefers to think of hot flashes as "her own personal summer... especially when having a flash in public!" Another Speaking of Women's Health presenter, Nancy Coey, refers to her hot flashes as "power surges!"

However you choose to view them, as your estrogen levels fall, your blood vessels open up and rapidly cause your skin temperature to rise. The feeling of a hot flash is a sudden sensation of heat in either your upper body or small of the back. It may move upward to your shoulders, neck and face. Some women report a prickly sensation in their face or body. You may become flushed and develop red blotches on your chest, neck, back and arms. You may start sweating... a lot. As the sweat begins to evaporate from your skin, you may become cold and shiver. Your "personal summer" moments can be mild or wake you from a deep sleep. They can last anywhere from 30 seconds to several minutes (even though it may feel like 30 seconds to 30 years).

Hot and Cold: Night sweats are often followed by chills. This cycle causes many women to have a hard time falling back to sleep. It may result in a restless night. Women reportedly wake up feeling tired because of this cycle. To help with insomnia, keep your bedroom cool to help prevent night sweats. In addition, exercise daily, but not just before bedtime.

Weight Gain and Sarcopenia: Many women lose muscle and gain weight during this transition. According to Dr. Michael Hewitt, sarcopenia (loss of muscle) may cause a lack of balance, resulting in a fall, and possibly a bone fracture. The most devastating fracture is a hip fracture.

While weight gain caused by heavier muscles is a positive; weight gain from body fat is a negative. It is true that the body's metabolism slows as we age. With a slower metabolism, many older Americans can also become more sedentary. Without proper exercise, the weight starts to slowly creep up on us.

Be careful about the weight you gain around your waist. It is known that people who carry excess weight around their middle (apple-shaped) are more susceptible to heart disease. See Chapters 3 and 4 – exercise and heart health.

Bone loss may become rapid during menopause. It is estimated that there is a 2% loss of bone per year for menopausal women. Think 2% is no big deal? Think again. Over the course of 10 years, you could lose more than 20% of your bone mass. To help protect yourself, see Chapter 5 for more information.

Emotional Changes: Irritability, moodiness, feeling down or depressed are common emotions during this transition. It is not clear if the emotional changes are due to hormones fluctuating or due to stress from family issues (aging parents, teenagers) or because of the lack of proper rest. There are studies that have stated that menopause does not cause depression, but the symptoms of depression may be heightened during this time in those who may have had underlying depression throughout their lives. To cope with mood swings, find a self-calming skill to practice, such as Yoga or meditation.

Problems with Concentration: Some women experience fatigue and diminished concentration as they approach menopause. These symptoms have, at times, been attributed to hormonal fluctuations. As with emotional changes, the stress of life may feed into concentration difficulties. More research is being done on cognitive changes that occur in women during menopause.

Vaginal Dryness: As estrogen levels decline, the tissues of the vagina and the external genitals often change. They can become drier, thinner, less elastic and somewhat delicate. The opening of the vagina may also become smaller and vaginal penetration can, therefore, be very uncomfortable. These changes are called atrophic vaginal changes and are a normal part of menopause for many women. Evelyn K. Resh, CNM, MPH, Director, Sexual Health Services at Canyon Ranch Health Resorts, encourages all peri- and post-menopausal women to use a water-soluble lubricant during sex. (It's best to avoid any petroleum-based products, as they can stay in the vagina for weeks and harbor bacteria). She also suggests that women who have moderate to severe symptoms discuss them with their health care provider and consider using vaginal estrogen on a regular basis. This form of estrogen is very safe and helpful for this problem and can make the difference between enjoying sex after menopause or avoiding it altogether due to pain. Check with your local pharmacist for the best products to use.

Sexual Desire: After menopause, your sex life isn't over! Many women report an increased satisfaction with sex once the risk of pregnancy is behind them and because they have more time with their partners now that their kids are grown. No matter what stage of life you're in, open communication about sex and feeling comfortable with your partner and your body are necessary for a satisfying sex life. If you have always enjoyed sex and then notice a significant decrease in your interest after menopause, check in with yourself. How are you feeling about your relationship?

Your Heart and Bones During Life's Transition.

✔ *Heart disease – Research has shown that estrogen bathes the heart and helps to keep it healthy. As we lose estrogen, we lose the protection that estrogen afforded us. After the age of 50, more women than men die of heart disease. Heart disease is the #1 killer of women. See Chapter 4 for more on heart disease.*

✔ *Osteoporosis – Losing estrogen causes women to begin to lose more bone than is replaced. This causes bones to become brittle and weak and they may break. Many women aren't even aware that they are at risk until a fracture occurs. See Chapter 5 for more information.*

How tired are you? And, how is your general health? Your answer to why you aren't enjoying sex may be found in the answers to these questions. If you feel that it would be helpful to seek counseling, make sure to find someone experienced in the field of sexual health who is comfortable talking about this subject. This will help you discuss it, too.

Skin: Collagen is in the skin and keeps it elastic, flexible and resilient. With declining levels of estrogen, there is a reduced amount of collagen found in the skin. This is the reason why the skin may become dry and wrinkled and look aged as women mature. In addition, our natural turnover of dead tissue cells slows, causing skin to appear dry, and soon, fine lines and wrinkles may appear.

Hair: Research has shown that hair follicles are also affected by estrogen loss. After menopause, some women may experience hair loss, a slower rate of hair growth, as well as a change in its texture.

Urinary Tract Symptoms: Normal urination or voiding occurs when the muscles around the urethra relax, the bladder contracts and urine streams from the bladder to the urethra and out of the body. As the bladder is emptied, the muscles around the urethra constrict, the bladder relaxes and the flow of urine stops.

Childbirth, aging and the lack of estrogen may cause the tissues that support the bladder and urethra to weaken. This problem can lead to urinary incontinence or symptoms of urgency and frequent urination. To help keep a healthy urinary tract, always drink plenty of water each day... or even consider cranberry juice!

Staying Healthy During and After Menopause
There is a link between menopause and a number of health problems that become more common as a woman ages. Understanding long-term health problems and learning how to reduce your risks can improve your overall health as you age.

Menopause does not have to be a silent passage... it should be a time to enjoy life to the fullest extent possible, looking forward to the years ahead. As time passes, so do our life's natural rhythms evolve. Take advantage of this time... you've earned it! Be sure to make your self a priority each and every day. Cherish the lessons learned and the wisdom gained. Rejoice in the grace, freedom, patience, wisdom and, most of all... humor that you've shared. Don't let life's transitions slow you down. Kick up your heels and ENJOY!

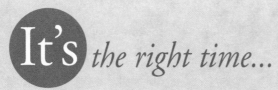

It's *the right time...*

To Learn About Your Options and Look Forward to the Years Ahead

Confused about what to do about hot flashes? Not sure if hormone replacement therapy is right or wrong for you? You're not alone! Evelyn K. Resh, Director, Sexual Health Services at Canyon Ranch Health Resorts provides the following information.

There has been so much controversy reported in the news over hormone replacement therapy (HRT) that women who are experiencing troubling symptoms of menopause are confused as to what to do. Just as there are benefits, there are also risks with hormone therapy.

For women with the following health issues, many health care providers advise against HRT:

✔ Breast cancer
✔ Endometrial cancer
✔ History of blood clots
✔ History of stroke
✔ Liver disease
✔ Abnormal vaginal bleeding

However, many agree that HRT is not wrong for every woman. If you have none of the health issues listed above, but are suffering from day-to-day, overwhelming symptoms of menopause, then short-term use of HRT may be a choice. For example, for relief from vaginal dryness, talk to your health care professional about vaginal tablets or topical estrogen creams that many experts feel are safe and effective.

Menopause is a time in your life when you and your health care provider have a special chance to work together and determine the best choice of action for your health.

www.speakingofwomenshealth.com

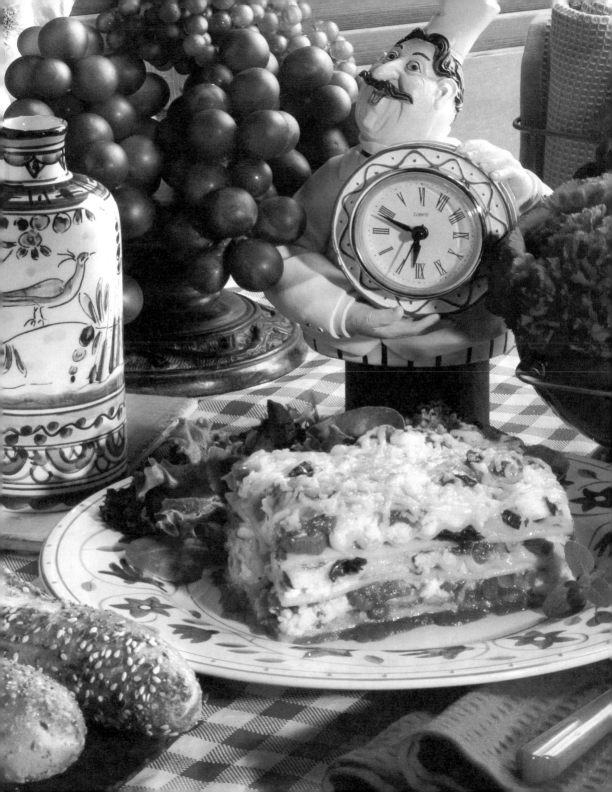

Veggie Lasagna

Thanks to Laurence R. Smith, II
Director of Marketing, HPV Franchise, Merck & Co., Inc.

Italians close their businesses for several hours each afternoon to enjoy a long, leisurely lunch, and then work late into the night. In the States, we take about 30 minutes for our lunch. Enjoy the best of both worlds... make this lasagna a day ahead and pack a serving to microwave for lunch.

INGREDIENTS

12	lasagna noodles, uncooked
2 medium	carrots, sliced diagonally
1 medium	onion, cut in half and each half sliced
1 cup	celery, thinly sliced fresh (or fennel)
1 medium	green bell pepper, seeded and sliced
1 Tbsp.	olive oil
	salt and pepper, to taste
1 medium	zucchini, sliced diagonally
1½ cups	spinach leaves, fresh
1 cup	sliced mushrooms, fresh
1	15 oz. container, part-skim ricotta cheese
1	egg
½ cup	grated Parmesan cheese, divided
1 cup	shredded mozzarella cheese, shredded
¼ cup	fresh basil, chopped
3 Tbsp.	chopped fresh parsley
4 cups	marinara sauce, jarred or homemade

NUTRITIONAL ANALYSIS
Servings per recipe: 8
Each serving contains approximately:

351	calories
18 g.	protein
45 g.	carbohydrates
11 g.	fat (5 g. saturated fat)

PREPARATION

- Preheat oven to 375 degrees. In a large pot of boiling, salted water, cook noodles until slightly chewy, about 8 minutes. Drain and carefully drape noodles over side of colander.

- While pasta boils, sauté carrots, onion, celery and bell pepper in skillet with olive oil. Sprinkle with salt and pepper, stirring frequently. When veggies are fork tender, add zucchini, spinach and mushrooms. Sauté until spinach wilts and all veggies are tender.

- In a small bowl, combine ricotta, egg, ¼ cup Parmesan, basil and parsley. Spray casserole dish with non-stick cooking spray.

- Spoon about ½ cup sauce into bottom of casserole dish. Reserve ¼ cup mozzarella. Arrange four noodles overlapping in casserole dish, top with about ⅓ the vegetable mixture, ⅓ the ricotta mixture, 1 cup sauce, ¼ cup mozzarella, and 1 Tbsp. Parmesan. Repeat, layering two more times, ending with sauce.

- Sprinkle top with remaining mozzarella, and bake 35–40 minutes until top is crusty.

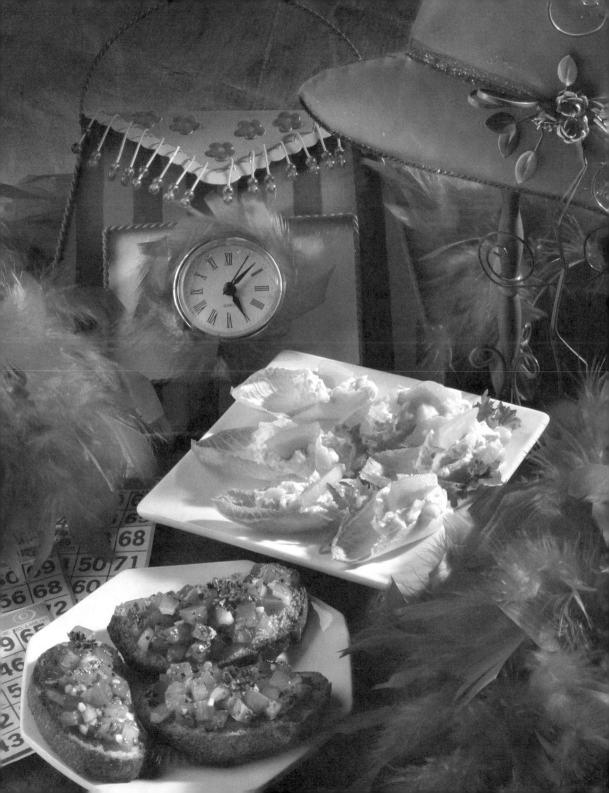

Healthy Appetizers

Thanks to Katie Taylor
Chief Customer Officer, Wal-Mart, Hanesbrands, Inc.

The poem goes: "When I grow old, I'll dress in purple and wear a red hat." Beat the clock and don't wait till you're older to be adventurous! Try your luck and serve some new appetizers... they're winners!

INGREDIENTS

Endive Mango Fig Appetizers

1	3 oz. package low-fat cream cheese, softened
¼ cup	coarsely chopped macadamia nuts
2–3	medium heads Belgian endive, separated into individual leaves
3	Calamyra figs, sliced
1	large mango or papaya, cut into thin strips (alternate choices include grapefruit sections, Mandarin oranges or pineapple chunks)
2 tsp.	lemon juice
¼ tsp.	lemon zest (orange will work also)

Bruschetta

2 large	tomatoes, coarsely chopped
2 Tbsp.	olive oil
2 tsp.	chopped fresh basil
½ loaf	Italian bread, cut into 1″ slices
¼ cup	freshly-grated Parmesan cheese

PREPARATION

Endive Mango Fig Appetizers

- In a small bowl, combine the cream cheese and macadamia nuts. Spread about 1 tsp. of the cream cheese mixture onto each endive leaf.
- Top with the mango strips, figs and other fruit choices. Arrange on a serving platter.

Make-Ahead Preparation

- Prepare as above through step 1. Loosely cover with plastic wrap; chill for up to 2 hours. Before serving, top with mango strips (or other fruit choices).

Bruschetta

- Preheat oven to 400 degrees.
- In a medium bowl, combine tomatoes, olive oil and basil. Place bread on a baking sheet, and top with tomato mixture. Sprinkle with Parmesan.
- Bake in preheated oven for 8–10 minutes, or until bottom of bread is browned. Allow to cool 5 minutes before serving.

For an additional healthy appetizer recipe, log on to www.speakingofwomenshealth.com and see our recipe for Salmon Spread.

NUTRITIONAL ANALYSIS – Bruschetta
Servings per recipe: 6
Each serving contains approximately:

178	calories
6 g.	protein
23 g.	carbohydrates
7 g.	fat

NUTRITIONAL ANALYSIS – Endive Mango Fig
Servings per recipe: about 24
Each serving contains approximately:

30	calories
9 g.	protein
2 g.	carbohydrates
2 g.	fat (1 g. saturated fat)

When Your Head Aches

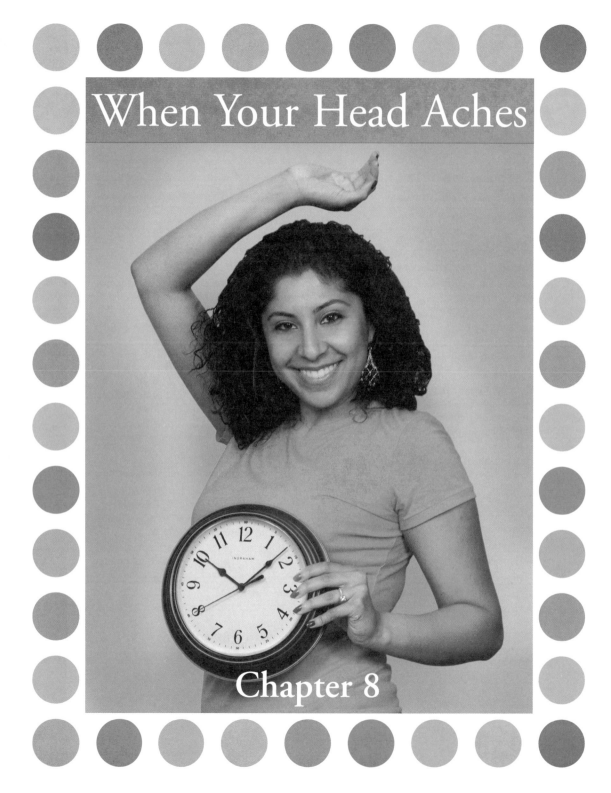

Chapter 8

HAVEN'T GOT TIME
FOR THE PAIN?...

Who Does?

There aren't many of us who can claim that we have never had a headache, or for that matter, not used that old familiar line... "Not tonight honey, I have a headache!" It is reported that 90% of us have experienced a headache. For millions of women, head pain is something that is all too familiar! *Headaches are not created equally.* The causes, as well as the severity and symptoms, may vary. The information in this chapter will aid you in understanding the different kinds of headaches and hopefully help you to see that you can be in control of your head pain and not allow it to control you!

Besides taking medication, try the following to ease the discomfort of a tension headache:

- *Take a warm shower or bath.*

- *Take a nap and make sure to get plenty of rest or sleep at night.*

- *Put a hot or cold pack on your head or neck.*

- *Take time away from the stress that is causing your headache. Go outside for some fresh air.*

- *Make exercise a part of your daily routine.*

Nearly half of the people in the United States who suffer from headaches do not seek treatment, and unfortunately, go undiagnosed and untreated.

If you experience any of the following symptoms, the National Headache Foundation suggests that you call your health care provider and schedule an appointment.

✔ Do you have several headaches per month, with each lasting for several hours?

✔ Do your headaches disrupt your home, work or school life?

✔ Do you have nausea, vomiting, vision or other sensory problems?

If you can answer "yes" to any one of these questions, then you need to take a moment out of your hectic schedule and think about what you need to do for yourself, your health and your well-being. **The good news is...** once a correct headache diagnosis is made, an effective treatment plan can be started.

What are the Different Types of Headaches?
Tension Headaches. The majority of headaches that most adults experience are classified as tension headaches. They are usually triggered by stress or anxiety and it typically causes pain felt all over the head. Many describe the feeling as a tight band of pain that encircles the skull. Usually starting in the middle of the day, tension headaches begin slowly and gradually build. Another name for this type of headache is a "stress headache." Whatever you choose to call your headaches, they are definitely a nuisance and can be mild to severe.

Tension headaches are caused from the tensing of muscles. When we are stressed, anxious, tired or overworked, the muscles in the face, neck, shoulders, back or scalp are all affected. Most of these types of headaches respond to over-the-counter remedies and are rarely due to a serious illness. If you have frequent headaches and nothing seems to be working for you, it is important to visit your health care provider. Together, you can determine a likely cause for your headaches and a proper course of action.

Take the time to tame a tension headache.

When stressed, we may unconsciously draw our shoulders up to our ears or grind our teeth or jaw without even recognizing that we are tense! Here are a few tips to remember:

✔ Take a few minutes during the day to relax your neck muscles.

✔ Take a slow, deep breath in through your nose, expanding your belly. Blow it out slowly, through your mouth, contracting your belly. It is amazing how a deep breath can help you feel relaxed. This breathing may also lower your blood pressure.

✔ Raise your shoulders up toward your ears, hold for a few seconds and then, let them drop. Feel the difference between the tension in your neck before you do this exercise, and how it feels when you release your shoulders.

The more you take time to recognize tension compared to relaxation, the more you will work toward keeping those muscles relaxed during your busy week!

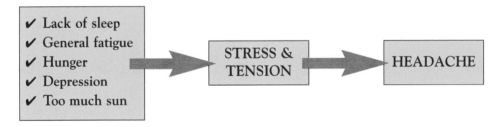

Migraines. Migraines affect 28 million Americans and women are said to be 4 times more likely to develop migraines than men. That equates to one in every 4 households having a migraine sufferer. More than just a bad headache, a migraine is a vascular headache. This means that it's likely the brain's blood vessels are constricting due to certain triggers. With this constriction, there is a diminished blood flow to the brain, which causes decreased oxygen supply. Reacting to the reduced oxygen supply, the brain's arteries dilate to meet the needs. This artery dilation triggers the release of pain-producing chemicals that irritate the nerves, thus producing the pain cycle.

Some Triggers for Headaches and Migraines

✔ Stress

✔ Emotional distress

✔ Not getting to bed and waking up at the same time every day

✔ Hormonal fluctuations

✔ Fatigue

✔ Weather changes

✔ Glare

✔ Dehydration

✔ Certain foods and lack of food

There are 2 categories of migraines, the **common** and the **classic** categories.

Common migraines are characterized by the following symptoms and may last hours, days or even weeks.

Migraines are:

✔ Usually one-sided, but can affect both sides of the head.

✔ Throbbing, intense pain – generally moderate to severe.

✔ Painful, felt near the eye of the affected side.

✔ Prone to cause nausea and vomiting.

✔ Often associated with sensitivity to noise or light.

A **classic migraine** is common among a group of sufferers who experience an "aura" or warning sign before the onset. It can include disturbing the sense of taste, smell or sound. The visual symptoms of flashing lights, spots or zigzag lines that can appear in one or both eyes are more common. Migraine sufferers may have blind spots or lose their vision for a short period of time. The aura can last 10–40 minutes and can be very frightening for the individual experiencing these symptoms. It is after this aura ends that the headache pain starts. Some sufferers experience no head discomfort, but have light sensitivity and feel tired.

Migraines are thought to be inherited. Talk with your family members about your family's history. It certainly helps to talk with others who are experiencing the same thing as you. Support from others can be a great source of comfort.

Migraine Facts
(Source: American Council for Headache Evaluation)

✔ Women are 3 times more likely than men to have migraine headaches.

✔ Migraine prevalence in women tends to peak between the ages of 35 and 45 years. This age bracket may be the time of raising children and building careers.

✔ Researchers are continuing to study the effect of hormonal fluctuations on headaches in women.

✔ 60% of women who suffer from migraines experience them during menstruation, in addition to other times of the month. 14% have migraines only during their menstrual period.

✔ Headache is one of the most common causes of absenteeism from work. On average, headache sufferers lose an average of 4 days per year. Women make nearly 10 million visits per year to their health care provider for headache evaluation.

Cluster Headaches. Headaches that occur again and again over a period of time are called cluster headaches. This type of headache is not as common in women as it is in men. Cluster headache sufferers typically experience a very severe shooting pain near one eye or temple. They have been frequently known as the "ice-pick headache," because of the severity. They seem to come in a series or succession for months at a time. It is for this reason that cluster headaches get their name. Another term used is "alarm clock headaches," because they may occur during sleep and wake a person at the same time each night.

Classified as a vascular type of headache, cluster headaches are believed to be connected with a lack of oxygen and dilated blood vessels. During a cluster headache, the person is quite often pacing, fidgeting or unable to sit still because of the intense discomfort. Other symptoms may include a stuffy or runny nose and a droopy eyelid over a red and tearing eye.

The cluster headache can last from 15 minutes to 3 hours. They can start at any age, but are usually seen beginning between the ages of 20 and 40. Unlike migraines, they do not tend to run in families.

Common Trigger Foods for Headaches and Migraines

✔ *Aged cheese*

✔ *Coffee/caffeine*

✔ *Nicotine*

✔ *Red wine*

✔ *Chocolate*

✔ *Asian foods with MSG*

✔ *Nitrates (in hot dogs and bacon)*

The location and type of pain has been compared to a "brain freeze" headache. We have all experienced one of these from eating ice cream too fast or drinking something ice cold too quickly. This analogy may bring insight to the experience of those who suffer from cluster headaches.

Medically speaking, cluster headaches are considered benign, meaning that they are not life-threatening. But, the fact remains, that the pain is so intense and severe that it is treated as a medical emergency by health care providers who understand the condition.

Because of the mysteriousness and intensity of the cluster headache, it has been misdiagnosed in the past. **You may want to talk to your pharmacist about suggestions for relief.** People with cluster headaches must be provided with effective and aggressive preventive and symptomatic relief measures.

Research has turned up several causes for cluster headaches, but unfortunately, no cures. Studies have shown that people with hazel eyes and heavy smokers are more likely to suffer from cluster headaches.

Triggers that often prompt cluster headaches include:
✔ Consumption of alcohol
✔ Strong smells (perfume or petroleum solvents)
✔ Heat, particularly for those with decreased tolerance to temperature fluctuations

The roles of diet and specific foods as triggers are controversial and not well understood.

Hormonal Headaches. Many researchers believe that changing hormone levels that occur during menstruation, pregnancy and menopause may be one of the reasons women have more headaches than men. The use of hormones (such as birth control pills) may trigger headaches in some women. Research is ongoing and will continue on the subject of women and hormones.

Sinus Headaches. You may have experienced a sinus headache, OUCH! A sudden move of the head or bending over is enough to bring the strongest person to his or her knees. Inflammation and pressure of the sinus cavities may cause constant pain in the forehead, cheekbones or across the nose. Triggers for a sinus headache may be allergies, due to the sinus congestion they cause, as well as colds or sinus infections. They may sometimes be mistaken for a migraine, because the pain may be as intense. You can treat sinus headaches with decongestants and analgesics. If over-the-counter medications are not working, contact your health care provider. An antibiotic may be prescribed if there is an infection involved.

Rebound Headaches. People who have chronic headaches may be taking medication 3 or more times a week. Over time, the medication may stop being effective in controlling the headache and in fact, may make it worse. This is called a "rebound headache." If you notice your medicine is no longer effective in treating your symptoms, it may be time to talk to your pharmacist or health care provider to discuss options available to break the cycle of this type of headache.

Goals for Controlling any Headache

There are two goals when treating any type of headache:

✔ Relieve the current pain

✔ Prevent future attacks

Make sure you avoid or minimize the causes or triggers of your headaches. Many headache sufferers tout the benefits of using relaxation techniques and other exercises. Prevention includes taking medications as prescribed. It may take a few weeks for the medications to work for you and there may be side effects. It is important to follow, as well as have patience with, your treatment plan.

It's *the right time...*
To Conquer Your Headaches
with Lifestyle Changes

You can take several steps that may very well help prevent your headaches. Review the following list and make some changes in your daily routines.

Identify stressors – Since day-to-day stress is one of the most common triggers for headaches, it is important to find healthier ways to deal with it. Think of ways to better cope with the stressors that you cannot avoid. Find ways of avoiding certain situations that you know will cause you stress. Make sure to take care of YOU.

Identify food triggers – Once you have determined the food culprits that may be triggering your headaches, make sure to carefully read all the labels of the food you purchase. You will be amazed at where you'll find some "trigger food" ingredients.

Adopt healthier eating habits – Make sure you choose foods that are healthy for you. Don't look at the changes as a "diet," but as a wise lifestyle choice that will allow you to feel better. Avoid letting too many hours pass between meals or skipping meals. This can cause chaos with your blood sugar and start a surge of hormonal changes in the body that can trigger a headache.

Something that is often overlooked is daily hydration. Not only is water important for your overall health, it is essential. Dehydration can be a trigger for many individuals, so keep a log of how many glasses of water you drink in a day.

"Work in" a "Workout" that is suitable for you on a daily basis – Regular exercise helps many women combat their tension headaches. Flexibility training is important, as well as strength-training. Both forms of exercise help with proper posture and may prevent muscle strain from occurring. You may remember relaxation tools you learned in childbirth or relaxation classes. These techniques work wonders in allowing you to recognize when you are tense and how to take a moment to relax those muscles. If you have a sitting job at work, get up, walk around and stretch from time to time. If you have a standing job, make sure you take a break and get off your feet.

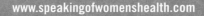

www.speakingofwomenshealth.com

Make sure to allow for some "Me Time" each day – As women, we all want what is best for our families and friends, and our jobs. Our personal concerns, however, are often put last or neglected altogether. We are all too familiar with this scenario, so it will take a conscious effort to make time each day for our own needs. It may be a walk in the park, taking time to read that book you never had a chance to enjoy, or buying your favorite magazine and creating a temporary relaxation area. Make this a priority every day. Pamper yourself!

Become better organized – Aren't there times that you just feel scattered and overwhelmed by every little detail of the day? Try getting yourself an organizational calendar. Making notes of the things you need to do for that day and crossing off the completed tasks can be very gratifying. This helps you make better use of the time you have.

Learn to say "yes" to yourself from time to time – How can you say "no" to the PTA when they ask you to be the secretary or "no" to the bake sale next week where you have to deliver 2 dozen cookies by 8 a.m.? Before you say "yes" to everybody else, be sure to say "yes" to "you" time.

Surround yourself with good friends and supportive family members – There is nothing more comforting than knowing that you can feel safe around your family or friends. If you have a headache, call them to help with the children or chores. Sometimes the hardest thing to do is to ask for the help that you need. Try it! You'll be surprised how many folks are willing to help you.

Time to take action! Many women just suffer through headaches, and in particular, migraines. If you've tried treating them with over-the-counter medications, and have made lifestyle adjustments to help prevent them AND, your life is still impacted by migraines... talk to your doctor. New medications that may help are available. Migraine prevention medication can help reduce the frequency of migraines. If that sounds like a new idea to you, it's because for most adults, daily migraine prevention medication is a whole new way to think about migraines.

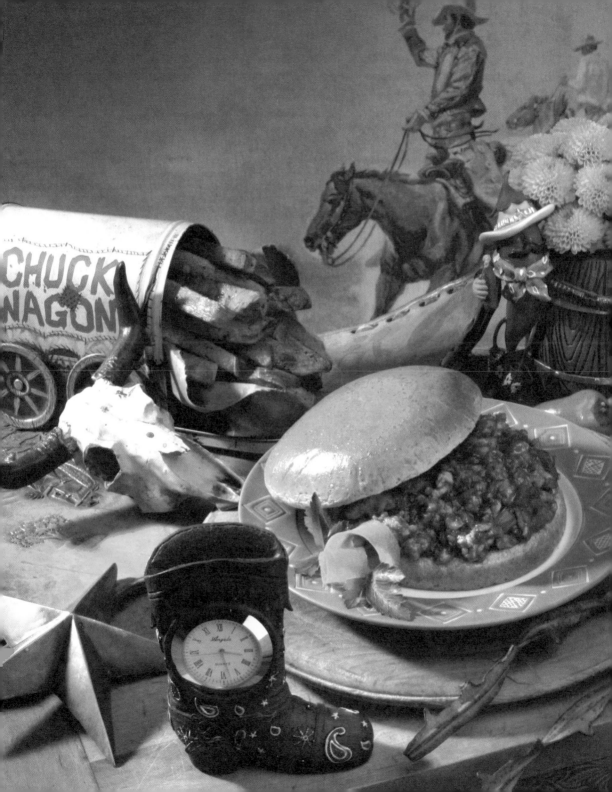

Healthy Joes and Oven Sweet Potato "Fries"

Thanks to Kelli Freeman
Vice President of Marketing, Cadbury Schweppes Americas Beverages

Bet your boots your friends will get a kick out of this new twist on an old favorite. Stake your claim with these sweet potato "fries" and neat sloppy joes. Just minutes from range to table.

INGREDIENTS

Healthy Joes

3/4 lb.	ground meat (*Turkey is best, or if you prefer beef, choose low-fat and rinse the meat after cooking. If you prefer, mix ½ ground turkey with ½ lean ground beef for added flavor. Lean beefs include ground round or chuck.*)
1 cup	onion, chopped
1	medium bell pepper, chopped
1½ cup	Ragu spaghetti sauce, meatless
3 Tbsp.	Hunts tomato paste
1	medium zucchini, shredded
1 Tbsp.	chili powder
1 tsp.	paprika
½ tsp.	garlic, minced
	salt and pepper, to taste
4	hamburger buns, whole wheat, split

Sweet Potato "Fries"

2 large	sweet potatoes, peeled and cut into wedges
½ tsp.	salt or salt-substitute
¼ tsp.	ground black pepper
	Optional: garlic powder, celery salt, seasoned salt

PREPARATION

Healthy Joes

- In large skillet, cook ground meat, onion and bell pepper over medium-high heat until meat is brown and onion is tender, about 7 minutes; stirring occasionally.
- Drain meat after cooking (rinse in colander under hot water if beef is used). Pat dry with a towel and return to skillet.
- Stir in spaghetti sauce, zucchini, chili powder, paprika, garlic, salt and pepper; bring to a boil over high heat.
- Reduce heat. Add tomato paste to thicken and simmer uncovered for 5 minutes.
- Spoon meat mixture onto buns.

Sweet Potato "Fries"

- Preheat oven to 400 degrees.
- Coat baking sheet with cooking spray.
- Arrange potato wedges on baking sheet in 1 layer and coat them with cooking spray. Sprinkle potatoes with salt or salt-substitute and black pepper, or optional seasonings. Roast 30 minutes, until tender and golden brown.

NUTRITIONAL ANALYSIS – Healthy Joes with bun
Servings per recipe: 4
Each serving contains approximately:

296	calories
26 g.	protein
18 g.	carbohydrates
14 g.	fat (3 g. saturated fat)

NUTRITIONAL ANALYSIS – Sweet Potato Fries
Servings per recipe: 4
Each serving contains approximately:

132	calories
1 g.	protein
16 g.	carbohydrates
7 g.	fat (1 g. saturated fat)

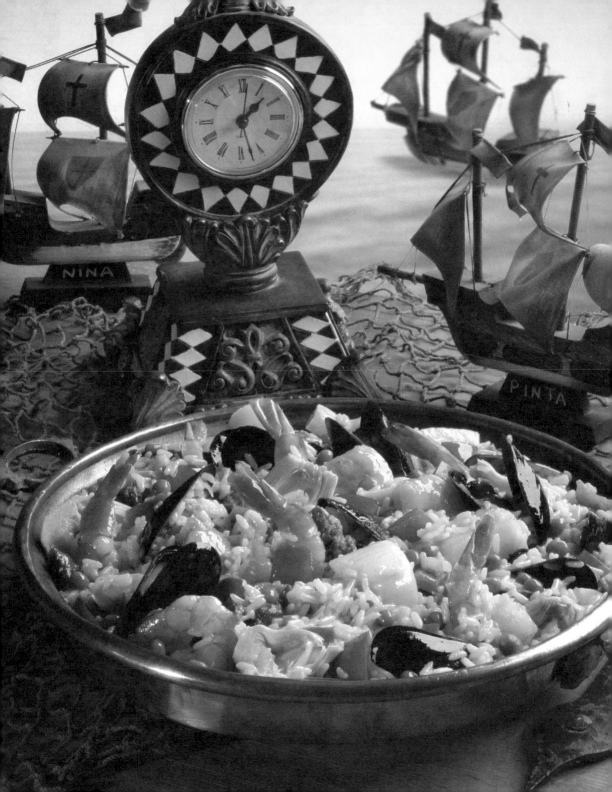

Spanish Paella

Thanks to Ana Fernandez
Manager, Customer Specific Marketing, Kellogg Company

Celebrate Columbus Day and set sail for a new world of healthy eating with this Spanish paella recipe. Queen Isabella knew when the time was right and so will you!

INGREDIENTS

1 lb.	seafood (choose from firm, mild fish cut into 1"–2" pieces; medium-size shrimp, peeled; scallops; crabmeat; mussels or small clams, de-bearded and scrubbed clean).

Seafood listed is a suggestion, but use whatever you like and is available. Experiment with different combinations for fun. However, DO NOT use oysters. Their unique taste clashes with the others.

½ lb.	chorizo or Italian sausage, (substitute turkey sausage to decrease fat)
3 Tbsp.	olive oil
1 medium	onion, chopped
1 medium	red bell pepper, cut into 1" slices
2-3	cloves garlic, minced or pressed
½ tsp.	paprika
½-1 tsp.	saffron, dissolved in ¼ cup hot water
	salt & pepper, to taste
1 large	tomato, finely chopped
1 cup	short-grain brown rice
1 can	artichoke hearts, drained
4 oz.	frozen peas, thawed
6 oz.	clam juice

PREPARATION

In a large, oven-proof skillet to be used for the sautéing, baking and serving:

- Sauté the sausage until cooked, if not already cooked. Remove the sausage, crumble and set aside. Wipe skillet clean.
- Sauté the onions, red pepper and garlic in the olive oil, until soft. Stir in the paprika, saffron liquid, salt and pepper.
- Preheat oven to 375 degrees. In 1" of water, steam clams and mussels until just opened, discard any clams or mussels that do not open. Remove with a slotted spoon. Combine the remaining water, the clam juice and enough water to make 4 cups of liquid. Bring to a boil.
- Add the tomatoes to the peppers, and sauté until hot. Stir in the uncooked rice and sauté 3–5 minutes. Add the hot clam juice and mix well. Cook over moderate heat, uncovered, for 5 minutes without stirring.
- Stir in the sausage and firm seafoods. Pat the ingredients into a flat, even, but still loose surface. Arrange the shrimp, scallops and artichokes. Press into the rice. Bake uncovered for 15 minutes, or until shrimp/scallops are just cooked.
- Arrange the clams and mussels, open side up, into the rice.
- Sprinkle the peas over the top. Bake for 5 more minutes.

NUTRITIONAL ANALYSIS
Servings per recipe: 6
Each serving contains approximately:

387	calories
25 g.	protein
36 g.	carbohydrates
16 g.	fat (5 g. saturated fat)

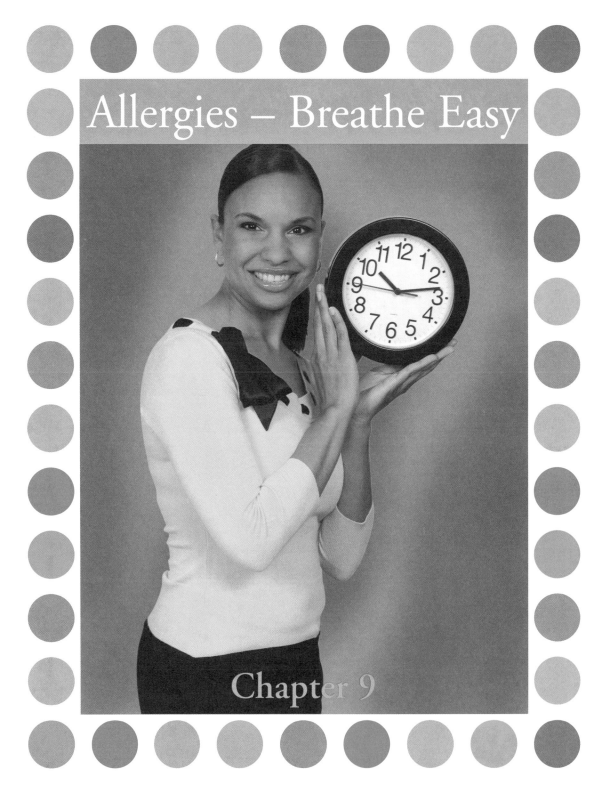

Allergies – Breathe Easy

Chapter 9

WINTER, SPRING, SUMMER OR FALL...

There's an allergy for them all!

The good news is... there are things you can do to prevent and control your allergies. The time is right to take a pledge to educate yourself about your options.

In this chapter, we will focus on what an allergy is, where allergies come from, as well as how to prevent and treat them. It's important to know that while allergies cannot be cured, there are numerous treatment options that can provide relief from the symptoms.

Allergies are extremely common; an estimated 40% of the population suffers from them. This leads to millions of missed work and school days annually.

What is an Allergy?

While this may seem hard to believe... an allergy is actually an over-reaction of your body's immune system. An allergic reaction is caused when the immune system reacts to certain substances that are usually harmless. These substances, called antigens or allergens, include food, dust, plant pollen and even some medicines. When the immune system identifies an antigen, it produces an antibody called immunoglobulin or IgE. This antibody causes the cells in the body to release a chemical called histamine. When the histamine kicks in, it creates itchy eyes, runny nose, skin irritation and difficulty breathing. When the same antigen presents itself again, the immune system restarts the process... thus causing another allergic reaction.

While the reactions are usually mild, at times they may become severe. An asthma attack is one example of a severe allergic reaction. It is often a reaction to something that has been breathed into the lungs of a person susceptible to that antigen. Another severe allergic reaction is called anaphylaxis. Signs of this reaction include difficulty breathing and swallowing, swelling of the lips, throat and tongue, dizziness and possible loss of consciousness. This reaction usually occurs within minutes of exposure to a trigger substance such as a peanut. Fortunately, these reactions do not occur often, and can be treated immediately with proper medical attention. Without the proper attention, anaphylaxis can be a very serious situation and even fatal. With this in mind, know your allergies!

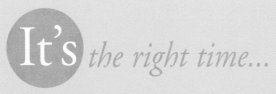
It's *the right time...*
To Conquer Your Allergies with Prevention

WHERE DO MY ALLERGIES COME FROM?

Often times, our allergies are hereditary and are passed down through the genes. While they may be passed down from a parent, a person usually does not inherit a single allergy, just the probability of having allergies.

Some of the most common allergic reactions result from:

Food – Any type of food can produce an allergic reaction. Most experts agree that the most common causes of food allergies are milk and other dairy products, eggs, soy, peanuts, tree nuts, shellfish, fish and wheat. Stomach cramps, vomiting and nausea are all symptoms of food allergies. Certain foods, such as peanuts and shellfish, can cause anaphylaxis, a condition that requires immediate medical attention.

Airborne Antigens – The most common types of allergies result from airborne particles. Typically, these allergic reactions are a result of the allergen being inhaled. Some examples of airborne antigens include pollen from trees and grasses, animal dander from pets, dust mites that live in homes, dust and mold.

Insect Stings – The poison from an insect sting can cause an allergic reaction. While most insect stings result in localized pain and swelling, people who are allergic to a particular poison from an insect bite can experience a severe reaction, including anaphylaxis. These severe reactions can occur very quickly and need immediate attention.

Medicines – The use of a certain antibiotic is the most common allergic reaction from medications. Always report any type of reaction from an antibiotic to your health care provider immediately. Allergic reactions from over-the-counter medications have also been reported. Again, if you experience any allergy-related symptoms from any medications, consult with your physician or pharmacist.

Chemicals – Standard household items, such as laundry soap and cleaners, can cause allergic skin reactions. Usually the chemicals in the products cause the reaction. Monitor your and your family's response to different items. Keep an updated list of the items that seem to cause a reaction.

Seasonal allergies such as hay fever are often triggered by pollen from plants, trees, grasses, etc. These symptoms can often be treated with over-the-counter antihistamines.

Treatment of Allergies

Seasonal allergies, like any chronic disease, play a role in weakening your body's immune system and increase your susceptibility to virus, which causes the common cold, among other things. Whatever the cause of your symptoms, the best treatment is to avoid contact with any substances that cause an allergic reaction. This means identifying the source of your troubles and avoiding contact. Frequent hand washing, a strengthened immune system through a healthy diet and daily activity and drinking plenty of water goes a long way toward the prevention of allergies.

Suggestions to help you avoid airborne allergies:

✔ Keep your windows and doors closed during peak pollen seasons.

✔ Always change your clothing after being outside and exposed to pollen.

✔ If dust mites cause a reaction, use special covers for your pillows and mattress.

✔ Keep pets out of certain rooms of the house, especially your bedroom.

✔ Consider hardwood floors, they do not accumulate as much dust as carpets and rugs.

✔ Clean your house frequently. A clean house with minimal dust is a great start.

✔ Always keep the air filter clean in your HVAC system.

✔ Wear a mask and gloves when using household cleaners.

While minimizing contact is the best way to avoid a reaction, other allergy treatments include medications and immunotherapy (allergy shots). There are several medications on the market used to treat allergies. The medications come as liquids, pills and nasal sprays. Even though these medications may help control various symptoms, they will not cure a specific allergy or reduce the likelihood of future reactions. For most allergies, an antihistamine is the usual medical treatment. At times, a decongestant is also recommended to help with a stuffy nose. There are antihistamine and decongestant combinations available to help relieve more than one allergy symptom. With all medications, always consult with your health care provider or pharmacist to determine the best course of action.

For those with potentially-severe allergic conditions, epinephrine is a fast-acting medication that can help with an anaphylactic reaction, which can be life-threatening. This self-administered injection comes in an easy-to-use container that is similar in size and shape to a writing pen. It is available only by prescription from your physician. These types of reactions usually require immediate medical attention. You may want to consider wearing an ID bracelet that states your allergic condition and contact information in case of an emergency.

Because several allergies cannot be avoided, especially airborne varieties, immunotherapy (allergy shots) is at times the best option. Immunotherapy is only prescribed for people with specific allergies and does not help with food allergies. Remember, the best treatment for food allergies is avoidance. Immunotherapy allows your body to slowly develop antibodies that help block future allergic reactions. While the thought of routine allergy shots seems troubling to some, they can be a highly-effective treatment for certain allergies. While injections do not cure the allergy, they do help increase the tolerance level when the body is exposed to the agent that causes the allergic reactions. This can lead to fewer reactions and milder symptoms. Consult with your health care provider if this type of treatment option seems appropriate.

If an allergy weakens your immune system, making you more susceptible to colds... here are a few tips to protect yourself and others.

✔ *Keep an instant hand sanitizer with you to kill germs.*

✔ *Drink plenty of fluids.*

✔ *Consider boosting your immune system with vitamins.*

✔ *To protect others, cover your mouth and nose when sneezing or coughing.*

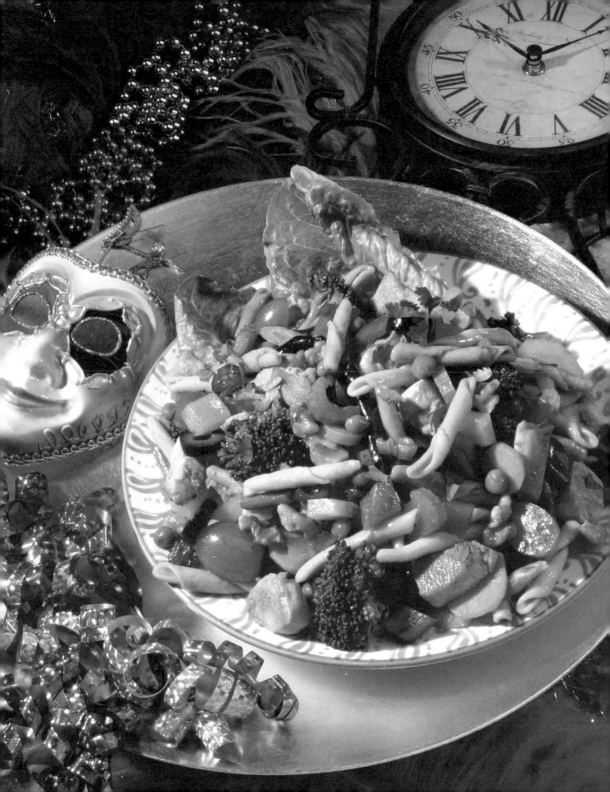

Mardi Gras Pasta Salad

Thanks to VeLois Bowers
Vice President, Diversity and Inclusion, Kellogg Company

Mardi Gras is a great time to celebrate, and this festive salad, made with tri-colored pasta, vibrant veggies and succulent chicken will set the mood. The Lenten clock begins at midnight... and this pasta salad (without the chicken) is a pretty Lenten option.

INGREDIENTS

1 lb.	tri-colored pasta (for a healthy alternative, try whole-wheat pasta)
1 cup	broccoli florets, fresh
2	boneless chicken breasts, cubed
2	celery stalks, sliced
2	carrots, sliced
½	red bell pepper, diced
½	yellow bell pepper, diced
¼	green bell pepper, diced
2	green onions (scallions) cut into pieces
8 oz.	shelled sweet peas, frozen or fresh
2 cups	fresh tomatoes (grape or cherry) cut in halves
8 oz. can	ripe olives, sliced
3-4 Tbsp.	cilantro
¾ cup	sesame seeds, toasted
½ cup	chopped walnuts
½ cup	dried cranberries
	Miss Ruth's All Natural Seasoning, to taste (no salt is preferred)
	raspberry vinegarette dressing as needed to coat pasta
2 Tbsp.	flaxseed
1	head Romaine lettuce to garnish the plate
3-4 Tbsp.	olive oil to sauté chicken breasts until tender

PREPARATION

- Cook pasta according to package directions.
- Sauté chicken in olive oil until juices run clear.
- Blanch the peas and set aside.
- Mix all ingredients together in a large bowl and toss.

Note: One pound of pasta (uncooked) will yield two to two-and-a-half pounds cooked pasta.

Provided with permission from Speaking of Women's Health speaker Chef Carmen Bazille.

NUTRITIONAL ANALYSIS
Servings per recipe: 6
Each 1 cup serving contains approximately:
- 409 calories
- 38 g. protein
- 35 g. carbohydrates
- 14 g. fat (2.5 g. saturated fat)

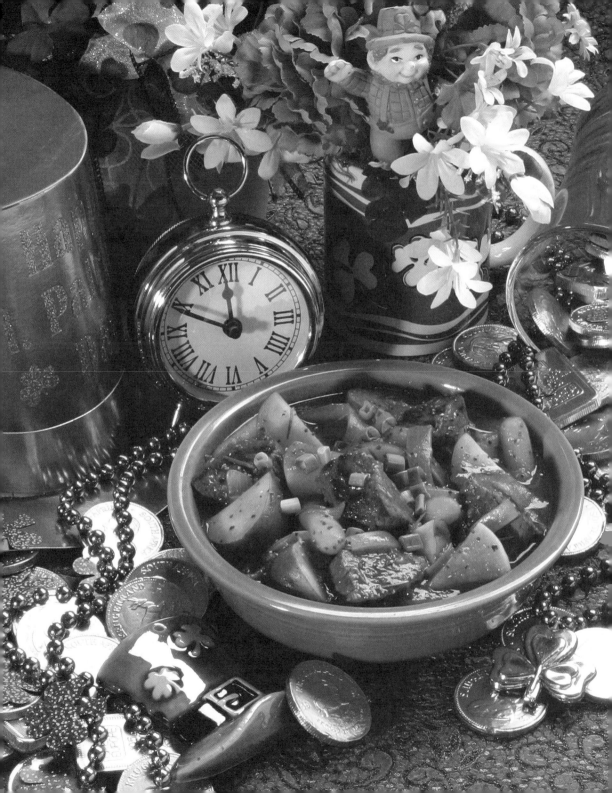

Irish Stout Stew

Thanks to Candace Matthews
President & General Manager, SoftSheen-Carson

With a little luck, you don't even have to be Irish to feed your family and guests this one-dish dinner. Make this delicious pot at the end of the rainbow and the raves will be golden!

INGREDIENTS

2 lbs.	lean stew beef (or lamb, if preferred)
1 clove	garlic, grated or ½ tsp. garlic powder
	salt and freshly ground black pepper, to taste
1 large	onion, halved and sliced
1-12 oz.	bottle Extra Stout beer
2 cups	beef broth (low-sodium)
3 Tbsp.	tomato paste
2 cups	baby carrots
4	new potatoes, cut into quarters
2	turnips, cut into quarters (if desired)
1	4-inch stem of rosemary, or 1 tsp. dried rosemary leaves
2	bay leaves
¼ cup	cornstarch
½ cup	water

PREPARATION

- Combine all ingredients (except the cornstarch and water) in a slow cooker and cook on low for 6-8 hours. Combine the cornstarch and water in a bowl and stir into the stew. Cover the slow cooker and allow the stew to cook an additional 10 minutes, until thickened slightly.

NUTRITIONAL ANALYSIS
Servings per recipe: 6
Each serving contains approximately:

385	calories
46 g.	protein
16 g.	carbohydrates
13 g.	fat (5 g. saturated fat)

Safety First

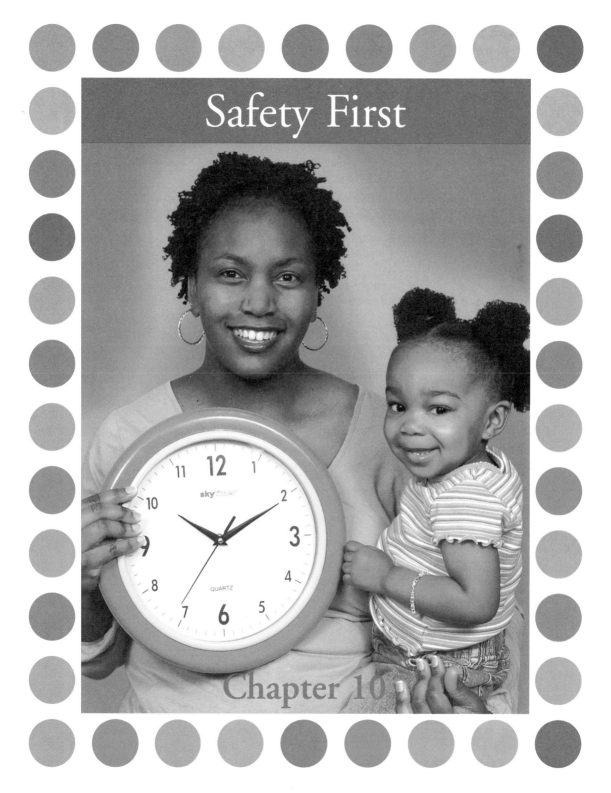

Chapter 10

SAFETY FIRST

It's the right time to get prepared for personal and family safety

Personal and family safety begins with learning what to do before you encounter an emergency. Whether it's an emergency as serious as to require CPR, or something as simple as treating bumps and bruises, today is the right time to equip your home with safety devices, a first-aid kit and an updated medicine cabinet, as well as a place to keep life-saving information, including your family's medical history.

This chapter is especially important this year as the CPR guidelines have been updated recently.

Safety at Home

According to the American Red Cross, fires are among the deadliest disasters to destroy homes across the country. Each year, nearly 5,000 Americans die in fires, and 80% of those deaths occur in home fires. Most residential fires are preventable.

Preparedness is your best weapon against deadly fires. Follow these simple steps to make your home "fire safe."

✔ Determine at least 2 ways to escape from every room of your home. Consider escape ladders for sleeping areas on the second or third floors. Learn how to use them and store them near the windows.

✔ Select a location outside your home where everyone would meet after escaping.

✔ Practice your escape plan at least twice a year by holding family fire drills. Experts know that even young children can save lives. Be certain your children understand the dangers of fire and how to get out of the home should one occur.

✔ When staying in hotels, make a game out of seeing who can locate the nearest fire exits when you arrive.

Follow these safety tips in the event that a fire strikes.

✔ Once you are out, stay out! Call the fire department from a neighbor's home.

✔ If you see smoke or fire in your first escape route, use your second way out. If you must exit through smoke, crawl low under the smoke to your exit. If you are escaping through a closed door, feel the door before opening it. If it is warm, use your second way out.

✔ If smoke, heat or flames block your exit routes, stay in the room with the door closed. Signal for help using a bright-colored cloth at the window. If there is a telephone in the room, call the fire department and tell them where you are.

*U*se *Your Head! Be Sure There's A Helmet On It!*

BE CERTAIN THAT YOUR CHILDREN WEAR A HELMET WHEN ON WHEELS, whether it's bikes, blades or skateboards! And, while you're at it… the best way to teach is by example. Make this a family rule!

It's *the right time...*

For Home Safety Prevention

✔ Equip your home with smoke and fire detectors, as well as a fire extinguisher in the kitchen, garage, workshop or other areas where fire may occur. Also, check the batteries in each detector twice a year. (NOTE: Be certain your home is free of carbon monoxide gases. At-home detectors are available.)

✔ Childproof your home, even if children are there just occasionally. This includes safety latches on cabinets and doors, closed doors near stairwells, childproof caps or a locked cabinet for medications, locked poisons and household detergents and child safety barriers for electrical outlets.

✔ Be sure all guns and firearms in your home or garage are stored in a locked cabinet. Store bullets in a separate, locked location and talk to children about gun safety at home and in others' homes.

✔ Teach children to practice safe habits around animals, even if they belong to someone they know. Animals can be unpredictable. Tell them to always ask permission from the owner before approaching an animal.

✔ Learn CPR and basic first aid, and require that regular babysitters take a basic first-aid class.

✔ Teach children to call 9-1-1 in the event of an emergency. (Even very young children can save lives.)

A Prescription for Safety... Don't Leave Home Without It!

The most important item to have in the event of a medical emergency is information. In the event of an emergency, when your emotions are at their peak, written and accurate information may save a life. Include:

✔ *Allergies. List any medication, food or latex allergies or sensitivities your family member may have.*

✔ *An updated list of your family's medications, including dosage.*

✔ *Any pre-existing illness or surgeries. Don't leave anything out. If a family member has a chronic condition such as diabetes, asthma or is allergic to medications, doctors suggest that they wear an identifying alert bracelet or necklace.*

Travel Safety

Whether your plans call for a week-long trip or just a day-trip by car, it pays to keep some simple safety tips in mind.

Traveling by car?

✔ Make sure your car is road-worthy before you start. Check oil level, the transmission fluid, the radiator's anti-freeze/coolant level, the windshield washer fluid, the brake fluid, the battery and all the cables.

✔ Remember to drive defensively and safely.

✔ Plan your route in advance and have a good map on hand.

✔ Keep your doors and trunk locked to protect your valuables.

✔ Always follow safety rules: use your seat belt, be sure children are properly secured in car seats, and always have a designated driver.

Once you arrive...

✔ Remain alert and aware of your surroundings at all times.

✔ Make note of exits and exit routes whenever you enter new places (hotels, restaurants, shopping malls, theaters, concert halls, etc.)

✔ Consider leaving expensive jewelry at home, or in the hotel's safe.

✔ Consider travel insurance.

R_x for safe travels

✔ If you are flying, keep your medications in your carry-on luggage, so that you have access to them during your flight and will not lose them in the event that your luggage gets lost. Plus, keeping your medications with you helps prevent exposure to extreme temperatures in the baggage compartment, which may alter a drug's effectiveness. Keep in mind, airport security requires that your medications be in their original, labeled containers.

✔ If your medication requires you to use a syringe (insulin, for instance) you may need to carry your prescription with you to ensure that you can pass through airport security.

✔ If you are traveling through several time zones, ask your pharmacist to work out a specific plan for adjusting the timing and dosage of your medications. This will prevent you from taking too much or too little.

✔ If you are visiting a hot, humid climate, be sure to keep your medications in a cool, dry place out of direct sunlight. Never store medications in the glove compartment of your car.

✔ Take along more medication than the number of days you've planned to be away. This will allow you to be prepared for unexpected delays.

First Aid Basics

If the last time you learned basic first aid was in grade school or high school, much of the information has not changed, but much is new, too.

The rise in the spread of blood-borne disease, including AIDS and hepatitis, has led to a whole new emphasis on protecting one's self from exposure to another person's blood or body fluids. Although the risk of contracting a disease is rare, according to the American Red Cross, the following precautions can reduce your risk:

1. Avoid contact with blood and other body fluids.

2. Use protective equipment, such as disposable gloves (available at any drug store) and breathing masks.

3. Thoroughly wash your hands with soap and water immediately after giving care to someone else.

If you do have to clean up a blood spill, do so immediately or as soon as possible after it occurs. Use disposable gloves and a breathing barrier, and wipe up the spill with paper towels or other absorbent material. Then flood the area with a solution of water and bleach (one gallon of water, $\frac{1}{4}$ cup bleach), allow it to stand for 20 minutes and then wipe it carefully. Throw away all material used in the cleanup in a labeled biohazard container.

First, Be Prepared!

Arm yourself with proper medicines and products to treat common injuries, ailments and illness. A well-stocked medicine cabinet is a good start.

According to the American Red Cross, a well-stocked cabinet should include:

- ✔ Adhesive bandages
- ✔ Adhesive tape
- ✔ Alcohol wipes
- ✔ Analgesic (relieves pain)
- ✔ Antacid (relieves upset stomach)
- ✔ Antibiotic ointment (reduces risk of infection)
- ✔ Antihistamine (relieves allergy symptoms)
- ✔ Mentholated chest rub
- ✔ Antiseptic (helps stop infection)
- ✔ Calibrated measuring spoon
- ✔ Disposable hot wrap and refreezable ice pack
- ✔ Decongestant (relieves stuffy nose and other cold symptoms)
- ✔ Disinfectant

- ✔ Fever reducer (adult and child). Do not give aspirin to children. Check with your pharmacist for a suitable substitute for reducing a child's fever.
- ✔ Gauze pads
- ✔ Hydrocortisone (relieves itching and inflammation)
- ✔ Syrup of ipecac (induces vomiting) and activated charcoal (absorbs poison, use when syrup of ipecac isn't recommended). Give syrup of ipecac or activated charcoal only after talking with your doctor or a Poison Control Center expert. Some ingested poisons are treated differently. *If you have a poisoning emergency, call 1-800-222-1222.*
- ✔ Thermometer
- ✔ Tweezers

First-Aid Kits

Be prepared away from home by keeping a first-aid kit on hand in the car, boat, barn, backpack or other convenient place. You can purchase kits, or assemble one yourself. Some kits are specifically created for particular activities like boating, hiking, etc.

Medicine Safety

According to Wal-Mart pharmacist Karen Froendhoff, some simple precautions will protect your family when taking medications.

✔ Remember that even over-the-counter medications and vitamins can cause serious problems, and even death, if a child or elderly person is overdosed.

✔ Only give family members medicines that have been prescribed specifically for them.

✔ Use the correct dose and read the label carefully.

✔ Follow the directions carefully, and do not confuse teaspoon (tsp.) with tablespoon (Tbsp.). If the medicine came with a measuring device, such as a dropper, medicine cup or dosing spoon, only use it and do not substitute another device when administering it to your child. A kitchen teaspoon is not appropriate for use in measuring medication.

✔ If a family member is already taking a medication, make sure that any other new medicines are compatible before combining.

✔ Consult your pharmacist about combining prescription medications with over-the-counter drugs, including vitamins and herbal supplements.

Inventory your medicine cabinet and first-aid kits at least once a year:

✔ Check expiration dates. Throw out all outdated medicine. If you're not sure about a certain item, call your pharmacist and ask what the shelf life of the medicine is.

✔ If medications are not in original containers or labeled clearly, throw them away. It's dangerous to store medicines in anything but their original containers. Some medicines come in tinted glass, for example, because exposure to light may cause deterioration.

✔ Every medication is a potential poison. If there are children in the house, keep all medicines and vitamins locked in a high cabinet, well out of reach.

Treating Shock: ABCs

No matter what the injury, someone administering first aid should always be on the lookout for shock. Shock means that the body has suffered a tremendous injury or trauma of some kind. Shock can be brought on by a severe injury, loss of blood, a life-threatening allergic reaction, poisoning or other event.

When shock occurs, the body's blood pressure drops suddenly, and the heart is not able to provide enough blood to the body's tissues. Signs of shock include:

✔ Restlessness or irritability

✔ Nausea and vomiting

✔ An altered level of consciousness (confused or dazed)

✔ Pale or ashen skin; cool or moist skin

✔ A blue tinge to the lips and fingernails

✔ Rapid or shallow breathing

✔ Rapid heartbeat

What to do if you suspect shock:

✔ Call 9-1-1

✔ Monitor the victim's **ABCs** – **A**irway, **B**reathing and **C**irculation

✔ Control any external bleeding

✔ Keep the victim from getting chilled or overheated

✔ Elevate the victim's legs about 8–12 inches, but only if you do not suspect a head, neck or back injury or that there are broken bones in the hips or legs.
   WARNING – If there is any chance of trauma or severe injury to the head, neck or spinal cord, never, ever attempt to move the victim. Moving the victim could further damage the spinal cord causing permanent paralysis or brain injury. The only exception to this rule is if the victim is under water. In this instance, bring the victim to the surface to enable breathing, taking care to support the head and neck as much as possible.

✔ Comfort and reassure the victim until advanced medical personnel arrive and take over. Do not give food or drink to someone in shock.

Controlling External Bleeding

If someone is bleeding, follow these steps:

✔ Put on disposable gloves to protect yourself.

✔ Cover the wound with a dressing (gauze or clean cloth) and press firmly and directly against the wound.

✔ Cover the wound by rolling it in gauze or a dressing, tear small strips at the end and tie a knot directly over the wound.

✔ If the bleeding does not stop, apply additional dressing and bandages. Apply pressure directly to the wound to squeeze the artery against the bone and call 9-1-1 or have someone near you call 9-1-1. Take steps to minimize shock.

CPR – Cardiopulmonary Resuscitation

CPR, or rescue breathing, is a form of intervention, usually administered to someone whose heart has stopped beating and who is no longer breathing. If only the breathing has stopped, rescue breathing alone can be administered to keep air flowing in and out of the lungs.

CPR is a two-stage approach in which the person providing first aid keeps pumping the victim's heart to keep blood flowing and blows air into the lungs to keep oxygen circulating through the body. It's always done until professional emergency medical help arrives.

The American Red Cross and others from the emergency response community recently created new guidelines for CPR in an effort to make CPR much simpler to administer, with the hope that simpler guidelines would encourage laypersons to use CPR, and specifically to administer chest compressions in an emergency.

First, Call 9-1-1 for Emergency Help.

To administer CPR:

First, lay the victim on his or her back. Place one or two hands in the center of the chest (on the lower-half of the sternum). Now place the heel of your first hand on top of the other hand, interlocking the fingers so that the fingers of bottom hand are raised off the victim's chest.

1. Give 30 compressions or downward thrusts. Position your shoulders over your hands and compress the chest – pushing downward – about two inches. Do 30 compressions in about 18 seconds, and keep the up-and-down movements smooth. Keep your hand in contact with the victim's chest at all times.

2. Now shift to the person's head and mouth to give rescue breaths. Open the person's airway by tilting the head backwards and lifting the chin. Pinch the victim's nose shut and seal your lips tightly around the person's mouth. Give 2 rescue breaths into the person's mouth, each lasting about 1 second. Watch the victim's chest rise to be sure your breaths go in.

3. Repeat the compression/breathing cycles.

4. CPR should not be interrupted or stopped until an AED (Automated External Defibrillator) is ready to use, another trained responder takes over or you see an obvious sign of life.

5. If the person has a pulse and is breathing, place the person in the recovery position (on his or her side), monitor the ABCs, and wait for emergency help to arrive.

6. If the person has a pulse, but still is not breathing, continue CPR. Wait for medical help to arrive.

7. If the person has no pulse and is not breathing, continue administering CPR – 30 compressions followed by 2 rescue breaths – until help arrives, or until you find signs of life.

IMPORTANT PHONE NUMBERS

EMERGENCY 9-1-1

Poison Control Center 1-800-222-1222

Police Department . . . . _____

Fire Department . . . . _____

Our Home Phone Number . . . . _____

Our Home Address: _____

_____

Dad's Work . . . . _____

Dad's Cell Phone . . . . _____

Mom's Work . . . . _____

Mom's Cell Phone . . . . _____

In Conclusion...

As you have read this book, we hope you have decided that "It's the Right Time" to take your pledge toward making informed decisions about your health, well-being and personal safety, not just for yourself... but for the health of your family, friends and loved ones. Small changes, done consistently, can improve the quality of your life and revitalize your spirit, at any age. Instead of counting the days... why not make ALL of your days count! And, live the new Speaking of Women's Health tagline every day: Be Strong - Be Healthy - Be In Charge. TAKE A PLEDGE FOR BETTER HEALTH at www.speakingofwomenshealth.com.

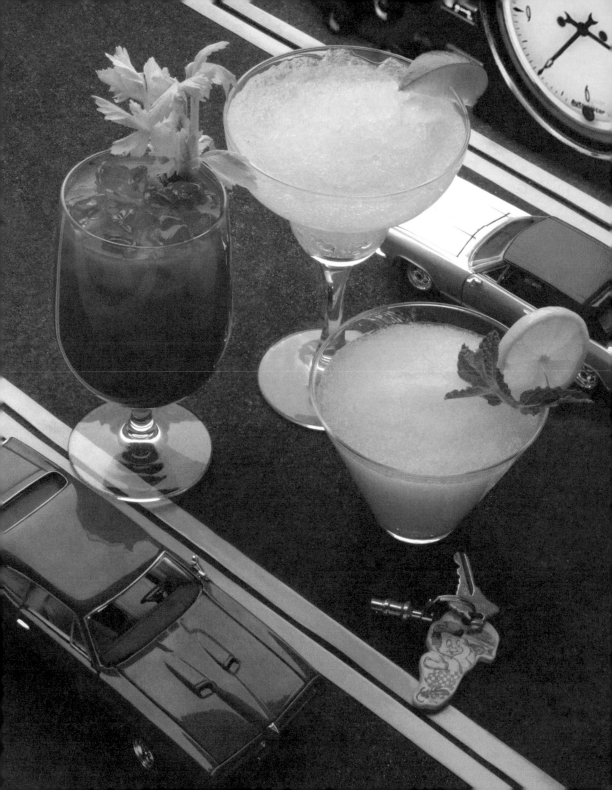

Mocktails

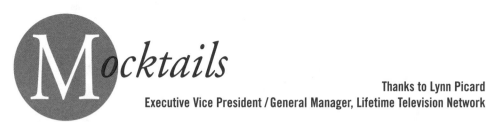

Thanks to Lynn Picard
Executive Vice President / General Manager, Lifetime Television Network

DON'T DRINK AND DRIVE...

The best time to pick a designated driver is before the party starts.
Serve these non-alcoholic mocktails and you and your guests can "party on!"
(With thanks to Canyon Ranch Health Resorts for this wonderful idea.)

INGREDIENTS

(Mock)-a-rita

2 oz.	lemonade or limeade, unreconstituted
8 oz.	cold water
½ oz.	lime juice, if using lemonade or lemon juice, if using limeade
6	ice cubes

PREPARATION

- Prepare in a blender on high for 10 seconds until light and frothy. Salt rim of margarita glass and fill.

NUTRITIONAL ANALYSIS
Servings per recipe: 2
Each 6 oz. serving contains approximately:
    53   calories
   14 g. carbohydrates

INGREDIENTS

Tomato (Mock)-tail

½ tsp.	Worcestershire
1 Tbsp.	lime (or lemon) juice
4 oz.	tomato or vegetable juice
	dash hot sauce (optional)
	salt, pepper and ice cubes

PREPARATION

- Stir in a mixing glass and pour over ice cubes. Strain off into a large cocktail glass.

NUTRITIONAL ANALYSIS
Servings per recipe: 1
Each 4 oz. serving contains approximately:
    27   calories
    1 g. protein
    7 g. carbohydrates

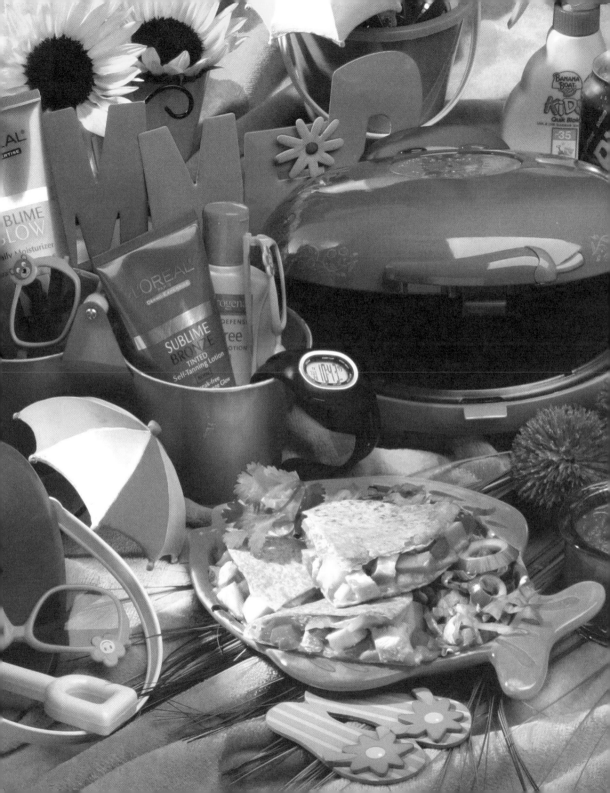

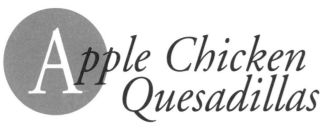

Apple Chicken Quesadillas

Thanks to Karen Fondu
President, Maybelline New York / Garnier

Watch your time in the sun... be smart and enjoy lunch in the shade. Try our quesadillas (with heart-healthy guacamole) and que sera, sera!

INGREDIENTS

2	medium, tart apples, sliced
1 cup	diced, cooked chicken breast
½ cup	shredded low-fat cheddar cheese
½ cup	shredded part-skim mozzarella cheese
½ cup	fresh or frozen corn, thawed
½ cup	chopped fresh tomatoes
½ cup	chopped onion
¼ tsp.	salt
6	whole-wheat flour tortillas (8 inches)
¾ cup	shredded lettuce
¾ cup	salsa (try fruity salsa for a sweeter taste)
6 Tbsp.	fat-free sour cream

PREPARATION

- Preheat oven to 400 degrees. In a bowl, combine the first 8 ingredients. Place about ¾ cup on half of each tortilla. Fold tortilla in half over filling and secure with toothpicks. Place on a baking sheet coated with non-stick cooking spray. Bake for 8–10 minutes or until golden brown.

- Carefully turn quesadillas over; bake 5–8 minutes longer or until golden. Discard toothpicks. Cut each quesadilla into three wedges; top with lettuce, salsa and sour cream.

NUTRITIONAL ANALYSIS
Servings per recipe: 6
Each serving contains approximately:

237	calories
20 g.	protein
19 g.	carbohydrates
10 g.	fat (5 g. saturated fat)

Index

OUR HOSPITAL PARTNERS*

Speaking of Women's Health is proud to partner with these hospitals to provide the latest, most up-to-date educational resources and information. As part of our mission to "educate women to make informed decisions about their health, well-being and personal safety," we have partnered with these health care institutions because we feel they have shared goals and a common vision with us.

St. Anthony Medical Center, Crown Point, IN

Manatee Memorial Lakewood Ranch, Sarasota, FL

The Women's Pavilion at St. Mark's Hospital, Salt Lake City, UT

Baptist Health, Jacksonville, FL

University Community Health and Tampa General Hospital, Tampa Bay, FL

St. Vincent Women's Hospital, Indianapolis, IN

Washington Regional Medical Center, Northwest AR

Shawnee Mission Medical Center, Kansas City, KS

Northwestern Memorial Hospital, Chicago, IL

WellStar Health System, Atlanta, GA

WakeMed Health & Hospitals, Raleigh, NC

Strong Health, Rochester, NY

Miami Valley Hospital, Dayton, OH

Cleveland Clinic Florida, Miami, FL

TriHealth Women's Health:
Bethesda North and Good Samaritan Hospitals, Cincinnati, OH

Boone Hospital, Columbia, MO

The Cleveland Clinic Foundation, Cleveland, OH

Sara Lee Center for Women's Health at Forsyth Medical Center, Winston-Salem, NC

King's Daughters' Hospital, Madison, IN

Margaret Mary Community Hospital, Batesville, IN

Covenant Health Systems, Waterloo, IA

Northwest Texas Health System, Amarillo, TX

Orlando Regional Healthcare, Orlando, FL

Sharpe Health Care System, San Diego, CA

Mercy Health Partners, Cincinnati, OH

Jackson Hospital, Montgomery, AL

Mills-Peninsula Health Services, San Mateo, CA

*as of this printing

Northwestern Memorial Hospital is delighted to partner with Speaking of Women's Health to provide the nutritional analysis through its Wellness Institute for the recipes featured in this book.

Building on more than a century of excellence in caring for women and their families, Northwestern's new Prentice Memorial Hospital will provide comprehensive health care for women throughout all stages of life. Prentice has long been recognized for excellence in obstetrics, the care of high-risk newborns and gynecology.

Opening in the fall of 2007, this state-of-the-art facility and its related women's health programs will support Northwestern's ongoing commitment to quality health care, with a vision to build on this strong foundation to make a lasting impact by setting the standard for what comprehensive women's health care can be. For more information on women's health, visit www.nmh.org.